*Welcome to **Nourishing Nephrons**, a cookbook crafted with care for those navigating the complexities of Chronic Kidney Disease (CKD) Stage 3. This book is more than just a collection of recipes; it's a comprehensive guide designed to empower individuals with Stage 3 CKD to take control of their health through nourishing, flavorful, and kidney-friendly meals.*

Chronic Kidney Disease is a serious health condition that affects millions worldwide, challenging individuals and their families with its dietary restrictions and lifestyle adjustments. However, managing Stage 3 CKD doesn't mean sacrificing taste or variety in your meals. With the right knowledge and culinary strategies, you can enjoy delicious dishes while supporting your kidney health.

In this cookbook, we've curated a wealth of nutrition strategies, culinary tips, and mouthwatering recipes specifically tailored for Stage 3 CKD. From breakfast to dinner, snacks to desserts, each recipe is meticulously crafted to align with the dietary guidelines recommended for CKD patients, focusing on limited sodium, potassium, and phosphorus content, while maximizing essential nutrients crucial for kidney health.

*Whether you're newly diagnosed or a seasoned CKD warrior, **Nourishing Nephrons** offers something for everyone. Discover the joy of cooking and eating well with recipes that are not only kidney-friendly but also tantalizing to the taste buds. From comforting classics to innovative culinary creations, embark on a journey to better health and culinary delight with *Nourishing Nephrons*.*

1. Oatmeal with blueberries and almond milk

Ingredients:
- 1/2 cup rolled oats
- 1 cup unsweetened almond milk
- 1/2 cup fresh or frozen blueberries
- 1 tsp honey (optional)

Instructions:
1. In a small saucepan, combine the rolled oats and almond milk.

2. Bring the mixture to a simmer over medium heat, stirring occasionally, until the oats are cooked and the mixture has thickened, about 5-7 minutes.

3. Remove from heat and stir in the blueberries.

4. If desired, drizzle with a small amount of honey for sweetness.

Nutritional Information:
- Calories: approximately 200 calories
- Protein: 5 grams
- Carbohydrates: 30 grams
- Fiber: 5 grams
- Sodium: low (depending on the type of oats and almond milk used)
- Potassium: moderate (blueberries are a good source)
- Phosphorus: moderate (oats and blueberries are moderate sources)

This recipe is a good option for individuals with chronic kidney disease stage 3 as it is low in sodium, moderate in potassium and phosphorus, and provides fiber and antioxidants from the blueberries. The almond milk is a dairy-free alternative that is also low in potassium. As always, it's important to consult with a healthcare provider or registered dietitian to ensure this recipe fits within your individual dietary needs.

2. Scrambled eggs with chives

Ingredients:
- 3 large eggs
- 1 tbsp low-fat milk or unsweetened almond milk
- 1 tbsp fresh chives, chopped
- 1/4 tsp salt (or to taste)
- 1/8 tsp ground black pepper

Instructions:
1. Crack the eggs into a small bowl and beat lightly with a fork. Add the milk and beat until well combined.

2. Stir in the chopped chives, salt, and pepper.

3. Coat a small non-stick skillet with cooking spray and heat over medium heat.

4. Pour the egg mixture into the skillet and let it sit for 20-30 seconds to set the bottom.

5. Using a spatula, gently push the cooked egg from the edges into the center, tilting the pan to allow the uncooked egg to flow to the edges.

6. Continue this process, gently folding and stirring the eggs, until they are softly scrambled and no longer runny, about 2-3 minutes total. Serve immediately.

Tips:
- Use low-fat or unsweetened milk to keep the potassium and phosphorus content lower.
- Chives are a good herb choice as they are low in potassium.
- Go easy on the salt, as sodium intake should be limited with kidney disease.
- Pair with a small portion of whole grain toast or a side of roasted vegetables for a balanced meal.

3. Apple cinnamon quinoa

Ingredients:
- 1 cup uncooked quinoa, rinsed
- 1 1/2 cups low-sodium vegetable or chicken broth
- 1 medium apple, peeled, cored and diced
- 1 tsp ground cinnamon
- 1/4 tsp ground nutmeg
- 1 tbsp honey or maple syrup (optional)
- 2 tbsp chopped walnuts (optional)

Instructions:

1. In a medium saucepan, combine the rinsed quinoa and broth. Bring to a boil over high heat.

2. Once boiling, reduce heat to low, cover and simmer for 15-20 minutes, until quinoa is tender and liquid is absorbed.

3. Remove from heat and fluff with a fork.

4. Stir in the diced apple, cinnamon, nutmeg and honey/maple syrup (if using).

5. Top with chopped walnuts, if desired.

Tips:

- Use low-sodium broth to keep sodium intake in check.
- Apples are a good fruit choice as they are lower in potassium.
- Cinnamon and nutmeg add flavor without needing extra salt.
- Walnuts provide healthy fats but can be omitted if needed.
- This makes a great breakfast or snack. Serve warm or chilled.

4. Low-sodium whole grain toast with avocado

Ingredients:
- 2 slices of low-sodium, low-phosphorus whole grain bread
- 1/2 ripe avocado, mashed
- Lemon juice (about 1 tsp)
- Ground black pepper to taste

Instructions:

1. Toast the low-sodium, low-phosphorus whole grain bread until lightly golden brown.

2. In a small bowl, mash the avocado and stir in the lemon juice.

3. Spread the avocado mixture evenly over the toast slices.

4. Season with a small amount of ground black pepper to taste.

Tips:

- Choose a bread that is specifically labeled as low in sodium and phosphorus, as these are important nutrients to limit with stage 3 chronic kidney disease.

- Lemon juice helps balance the creaminess of the avocado without adding extra salt.

- Avoid adding any additional salt, as sodium intake should be restricted.

- Pair this with other low-sodium, low-phosphorus foods for a kidney-friendly meal or snack.

This recipe provides healthy fats, fiber, and nutrients while keeping sodium and phosphorus levels in check for someone with stage 3 chronic kidney disease. The avocado provides creaminess and healthy monounsaturated fats.

5. Smoothie with mixed berries, spinach, and water

Ingredients:
- 1 cup mixed berries (such as blueberries, raspberries, and blackberries)
- 1 cup fresh spinach leaves
- 1 cup water

Instructions:
1. Add the mixed berries, spinach leaves, and water to a blender.

2. Blend on high speed until smooth and creamy.

Tips:
- Choose a variety of low-potassium berries like blueberries, raspberries, and blackberries. Avoid high-potassium fruits like bananas.

- Spinach is a good source of nutrients while being relatively low in potassium compared to other greens.

- Use water instead of milk or juice to keep the smoothie low in phosphorus and potassium.
- Adjust the amount of water to reach your desired consistency.

- Avoid adding any other ingredients like yogurt, protein powder, or sweeteners, as these may be high in phosphorus or potassium.

This smoothie provides a nutrient-dense, low-potassium, and low-phosphorus option for someone with stage 3 chronic kidney disease. The berries and spinach offer antioxidants, fiber, and other beneficial nutrients without overloading the kidneys.

6. Greek yogurt with strawberries

Ingredients:
- 1 cup low-fat, low-sodium Greek yogurt
- 1 cup fresh strawberries, sliced

Instructions:
1. Spoon the Greek yogurt into a bowl.

2. Top the yogurt with the sliced strawberries.

Tips:

- Choose a low-fat, low-sodium Greek yogurt to keep the phosphorus and sodium content low.

- Strawberries are a good choice of fruit as they are relatively low in potassium compared to many other fruits.

- Avoid adding any other toppings or sweeteners, as these may be high in phosphorus, potassium, or sodium.

- You can also use other low-potassium berries like blueberries or raspberries instead of strawberries.

- This makes a simple, nutrient-dense snack or light meal that is kidney-friendly.

This combination of low-fat Greek yogurt and fresh strawberries provides protein, calcium, and other beneficial nutrients, while keeping the potassium, phosphorus, and sodium content in check for someone with stage 3 chronic kidney disease.

7. Cottage cheese with pineapple

Ingredients:
- 1 cup low-fat, low-sodium cottage cheese
- 1/2 cup fresh pineapple, diced

Instructions:
1. Spoon the cottage cheese into a bowl.

2. Top the cottage cheese with the diced pineapple.

Tips:
- Choose a low-fat, low-sodium cottage cheese to keep the phosphorus and sodium content low.

- Pineapple is a good choice of fruit as it is relatively low in potassium compared to many other fruits.

- Avoid adding any other toppings or sweeteners, as these may be high in phosphorus, potassium, or sodium.

- You can also use other low-potassium fruits like blueberries or mandarin oranges instead of pineapple.

- This makes a simple, nutrient-dense snack or light meal that is kidney-friendly.

This combination of low-fat cottage cheese and fresh pineapple provides protein, calcium, and other beneficial nutrients, while keeping the potassium, phosphorus, and sodium content in check for someone with stage 3 chronic kidney disease.

8. Banana pancakes (using almond flour)

Ingredients:
- 1 ripe banana, mashed
- 2 eggs
- 1/4 cup almond flour
- 1/4 tsp baking powder
- 1/4 tsp ground cinnamon (optional)
- Cooking spray or oil (such as olive oil)

Instructions:
1. In a medium bowl, mash the ripe banana until smooth.

2. Add the eggs and whisk together until well combined.

3. Stir in the almond flour, baking powder, and cinnamon (if using) until a smooth batter forms.

4. Heat a non-stick skillet or griddle over medium heat and lightly coat with cooking spray or oil.

5. Scoop the batter onto the hot surface, forming pancakes about 3-4 inches in diameter.

6. Cook for 2-3 minutes per side, or until golden brown.

7. Serve the banana pancakes warm.

Tips:
- Almond flour is a low-potassium, low-phosphorus flour option for those with chronic kidney disease.

- Bananas are high in potassium, so this recipe uses just one ripe banana to limit the potassium content.

- Avoid adding any additional toppings or syrups, as these may be high in phosphorus or potassium.

- Serve the pancakes plain or with a small amount of low-fat, low-sodium cottage cheese or Greek yogurt.

These banana pancakes made with almond flour provide a kidney-friendly, nutrient-dense breakfast option for those with stage 3 chronic kidney disease.

9. Rice cakes with peanut butter

Ingredients:
- 2 low-sodium, low-phosphorus rice cakes
- 2 tbsp natural, unsalted peanut butter

Instructions: 1. Spread the peanut butter evenly over the rice cakes.

Tips:
- Choose rice cakes that are specifically labeled as low in sodium and phosphorus, as these are important nutrients to limit with stage 3 chronic kidney disease.

- Use a natural, unsalted peanut butter to keep the sodium content low.

- Avoid adding any additional toppings or sweeteners, as these may be high in phosphorus, potassium, or sodium.

- This makes a simple, portable snack that provides protein and healthy fats.

This combination of low-sodium, low-phosphorus rice cakes and natural peanut butter provides a nutrient-dense, kidney-friendly option for someone with stage 3 chronic kidney disease. The peanut butter offers protein and healthy fats, while the rice cakes provide a low-potassium carbohydrate source.

Remember, it's important to consult with a registered dietitian or your healthcare provider to ensure your dietary needs are being met while managing chronic kidney disease.

10. Egg white omelet with bell peppers

Ingredients:
- 3 egg whites
- 1/4 cup diced bell peppers (any color)
- 1 tsp olive oil
- Salt and pepper to taste (use very little salt)

Instructions:
1. In a small bowl, whisk the egg whites until frothy.

2. Heat the olive oil in a non-stick skillet over medium heat.

3. Pour the egg whites into the skillet and let them cook for 1-2 minutes.

4. Sprinkle the diced bell peppers over the top of the egg whites.

5. Use a spatula to gently fold the omelet in half and slide it onto a plate.

6. Season with a small amount of salt and pepper to taste.

Tips:
- Egg whites are a good source of protein while being low in phosphorus compared to whole eggs.

- Bell peppers are a low-potassium vegetable that adds flavor and nutrients to the omelet.

- Use just a small amount of salt, as sodium intake should be limited with stage 3 chronic kidney disease.

- Avoid adding any other fillings or toppings that may be high in potassium, phosphorus, or sodium.

- Serve the omelet with a side of low-sodium, low-phosphorus toast or a small portion of low-potassium fruit.

This egg white omelet with bell peppers provides a nutrient-dense, kidney-friendly breakfast or snack option for someone with stage 3 chronic kidney disease.

11. Grilled chicken salad with mixed greens

Ingredients:
- 4 oz grilled chicken breast, sliced
- 2 cups mixed greens (such as spinach, romaine, and arugula)
- 1/2 cup diced cucumber
- 1/4 cup diced tomatoes
- 1 tbsp olive oil
- 1 tbsp balsamic vinegar
- Salt and pepper to taste (use very little salt)

Instructions:

1. In a large salad bowl, combine the mixed greens, diced cucumber, and diced tomatoes.

2. Top the salad with the sliced grilled chicken.

3. Drizzle the olive oil and balsamic vinegar over the salad.

4. Season with a small amount of salt and pepper to taste.

Tips:

- Choose a lean protein source like grilled chicken breast to keep the phosphorus and sodium content low.

- Mixed greens like spinach, romaine, and arugula are low in potassium compared to other greens.

- Cucumber and tomatoes are also low-potassium vegetables that add flavor and nutrients to the salad.

- Use a simple dressing of olive oil and balsamic vinegar to avoid high-sodium or high-phosphorus dressings.

- Avoid adding any other toppings or ingredients that may be high in potassium, phosphorus, or sodium.

This grilled chicken salad with mixed greens provides a nutrient-dense, kidney-friendly meal option for someone with stage 3 chronic kidney disease. The combination of lean protein, low-potassium vegetables, and a simple dressing makes it a balanced and satisfying option.

12. Quinoa and vegetable stir-fry

Ingredients:
- 1/2 cup cooked quinoa
- 1 tbsp olive oil
- 1/2 cup diced bell peppers
- 1/2 cup diced zucchini
- 1/4 cup diced onion
- 1 clove garlic, minced
- 2 tbsp low-sodium soy sauce or tamari
- Salt and pepper to taste (use very little salt)

Instructions:
1. Cook the quinoa according to package instructions. Set aside.

2. In a large skillet or wok, heat the olive oil over medium-high heat.

3. Add the diced bell peppers, zucchini, onion, and garlic. Stir-fry for 5-7 minutes, until the vegetables are tender-crisp.

4. Add the cooked quinoa and low-sodium soy sauce or tamari. Stir to combine and heat through.

5. Season with a small amount of salt and pepper to taste.

Tips:
- Quinoa is a low-potassium, low-phosphorus grain that provides fiber and protein.

- Choose a variety of low-potassium vegetables like bell peppers, zucchini, and onions.

- Use low-sodium soy sauce or tamari to keep the sodium content in check.

- Avoid adding any other high-potassium or high-phosphorus ingredients.

- Serve the stir-fry as a main dish or pair it with a small portion of a low-potassium fruit.

This quinoa and vegetable stir-fry provides a nutrient-dense, kidney-friendly meal option for someone with stage 3 chronic kidney disease. The combination of quinoa, vegetables, and a simple soy-based sauce makes it a flavorful and satisfying dish.

13. Tuna salad with cucumber and dill (using Greek yogurt)

Ingredients:
- 1 (5 oz) can of water-packed tuna, drained
- 1/4 cup plain, low-fat Greek yogurt
- 1/4 cup diced cucumber
- 1 tbsp chopped fresh dill
- 1 tsp lemon juice
- Salt and pepper to taste (use very little salt)

Instructions:
1. In a medium bowl, combine the drained tuna, Greek yogurt, diced cucumber, chopped dill, and lemon juice.

2. Gently mix all the ingredients together until well combined.

3. Season with a small amount of salt and pepper to taste.

Tips:
- Choose water-packed tuna to keep the sodium content low.

- Greek yogurt provides a creamy texture while being lower in phosphorus than mayonnaise.

- Cucumber is a low-potassium vegetable that adds crunch and flavor.

- Fresh dill adds a nice herbal note without adding extra sodium or potassium.

- Lemon juice helps balance the flavors without needing to add salt.

- Serve the tuna salad on a bed of mixed greens, on a slice of low-sodium, low-phosphorus toast, or with a side of sliced cucumber.

This tuna salad with Greek yogurt, cucumber, and dill makes a nutrient-dense, kidney-friendly snack or light meal for someone with stage 3 chronic kidney disease. The combination of protein, low-potassium vegetables, and a simple dressing provides a flavorful and satisfying option.

14. Lentil soup with carrots and celery

Ingredients:
- 1 cup dry brown or green lentils, rinsed
- 4 cups low-sodium vegetable or chicken broth
- 1 cup diced carrots
- 1 cup diced celery
- 1 small onion, diced
- 2 cloves garlic, minced
- 1 tsp dried thyme
- Salt and pepper to taste (use very little salt)

Instructions:
1. In a large pot, combine the rinsed lentils and broth. Bring to a boil over high heat.

2. Once boiling, reduce heat to medium-low and let the lentils simmer for 15-20 minutes, until tender.

3. Add the diced carrots, celery, onion, and garlic to the pot. Simmer for an additional 10-15 minutes, until the vegetables are tender.

4. Stir in the dried thyme and season with a small amount of salt and pepper to taste.

Tips:
- Lentils are a great source of protein and fiber while being low in phosphorus.

- Carrots and celery are low-potassium vegetables that add flavor and nutrients to the soup.
- Use a low-sodium broth to keep the sodium content in check.

- Avoid adding any high-potassium vegetables or ingredients that may be high in phosphorus.

- Serve the lentil soup on its own or with a small side salad of mixed greens.

This lentil soup with carrots and celery provides a nutrient-dense, kidney-friendly meal option for someone with stage 3 chronic kidney disease. The combination of protein-rich lentils and low-potassium vegetables makes it a satisfying and healthy choice.

15. Turkey and avocado wrap (using whole grain tortilla)

Ingredients:
- 1 (8-inch) whole grain tortilla, low in sodium and phosphorus
- 2-3 oz sliced turkey breast
- 1/2 ripe avocado, sliced
- 1 tbsp low-fat, low-sodium cream cheese
- 1 tbsp diced tomatoes
- Salt and pepper to taste (use very little salt)

Instructions:
1. Lay the whole grain tortilla flat on a clean surface.

2. Spread the low-fat, low-sodium cream cheese evenly over the tortilla.

3. Layer the sliced turkey breast, avocado slices, and diced tomatoes on top of the cream cheese.

4. Season with a small amount of salt and pepper to taste.

5. Carefully roll up the tortilla, tucking in the sides as you go, to create a wrap.

Tips:
- Choose a whole grain tortilla that is specifically labeled as low in sodium and phosphorus.
- Turkey breast is a lean protein source that is low in phosphorus.

- Avocado provides healthy fats and creaminess without adding extra sodium or potassium.
- Tomatoes are a low-potassium vegetable that adds flavor.

- Avoid adding any other high-sodium, high-potassium, or high-phosphorus ingredients.

- You can also serve the wrap with a side of raw, low-potassium vegetables like cucumber or bell peppers.

This turkey and avocado wrap with a whole grain tortilla makes a nutrient-dense, kidney-friendly lunch or snack option for someone with stage 3 chronic kidney disease. The combination of lean protein, healthy fats, and low-potassium vegetables provides a balanced and satisfying meal.

16. Mixed greens with apples, walnuts, and vinaigrette

Ingredients:
- 2 cups mixed greens (such as spinach, arugula, and romaine)
- 1/2 cup diced apples (such as Gala or Fuji)
- 2 tbsp chopped walnuts
- 1 tbsp olive oil
- 1 tbsp balsamic vinegar
- Salt and pepper to taste (use very little salt)

Instructions:
1. In a large salad bowl, combine the mixed greens, diced apples, and chopped walnuts.

2. In a small bowl, whisk together the olive oil and balsamic vinegar to make the vinaigrette.

3. Drizzle the vinaigrette over the salad and toss gently to coat.

4. Season with a small amount of salt and pepper to taste.

Tips:
- Choose a variety of low-potassium greens like spinach, arugula, and romaine.

- Apples are a low-potassium fruit that adds sweetness and crunch to the salad.

- Walnuts provide healthy fats and a satisfying crunch, while being low in phosphorus.

- The simple vinaigrette of olive oil and balsamic vinegar keeps the sodium and phosphorus content low.

- Avoid adding any other high-potassium or high-phosphorus toppings or dressings.

- This salad can be served as a side dish or a light main course.

This mixed greens salad with apples, walnuts, and a balsamic vinaigrette provides a nutrient-dense, kidney-friendly option for someone with stage 3 chronic kidney disease. The combination of low-potassium greens, fruit, and healthy fats makes it a balanced and flavorful choice.

17. Low-sodium turkey and cheese sandwich

Ingredients:
- 2 slices of low-sodium, low-phosphorus whole grain bread
- 2-3 oz sliced low-sodium turkey breast
- 1 slice of low-fat, low-sodium cheese (such as cheddar or Swiss)
- Lettuce leaves (optional)
- Tomato slices (optional)
- Mustard or mayonnaise (optional, use low-sodium versions)

Instructions:
1. Place one slice of the low-sodium, low-phosphorus whole grain bread on a clean surface.

2. Layer the sliced low-sodium turkey breast on top of the bread.

3. Top the turkey with the slice of low-fat, low-sodium cheese.

4. If desired, add a few lettuce leaves and tomato slices.

5. Spread a small amount of low-sodium mustard or mayonnaise on the second slice of bread, if using.

6. Place the second slice of bread on top to complete the sandwich.

Tips:
- Choose a whole grain bread that is specifically labeled as low in sodium and phosphorus.

- Look for low-sodium turkey breast and low-fat, low-sodium cheese to keep the sodium and phosphorus content in check.

- Lettuce and tomato are low-potassium vegetables that can add flavor and crunch.

- Use only a small amount of low-sodium condiments like mustard or mayonnaise, as these can also be high in sodium.

- Avoid adding any other high-sodium, high-potassium, or high-phosphorus ingredients.

- Serve the sandwich with a side of raw, low-potassium vegetables or a small piece of low-potassium fruit.

This low-sodium turkey and cheese sandwich provides a simple, nutrient-dense, and kidney-friendly option for someone with stage 3 chronic kidney disease.

18. Spinach and strawberry salad with poppy seed dressing

Ingredients:
Salad:
- 2 cups fresh spinach leaves
- 1 cup sliced fresh strawberries
- 2 tbsp chopped walnuts

Poppy Seed Dressing:
- 2 tbsp olive oil
- 1 tbsp white wine vinegar
- 1 tsp Dijon mustard
- 1 tsp honey
- 1 tsp poppy seeds
- Salt and pepper to taste (use very little salt)

Instructions:
1. In a large salad bowl, combine the spinach leaves, sliced strawberries, and chopped walnuts.

2. In a small bowl, whisk together the olive oil, white wine vinegar, Dijon mustard, honey, and poppy seeds to make the dressing.

3. Drizzle the poppy seed dressing over the salad and toss gently to coat.

4. Season with a small amount of salt and pepper to taste.

Tips:
- Spinach is a low-potassium green that provides nutrients without overloading the kidneys.

- Strawberries are a low-potassium fruit that adds sweetness and color to the salad.

- Walnuts are a good source of healthy fats while being low in phosphorus.

- The simple poppy seed dressing uses minimal ingredients to keep the sodium and phosphorus content low.

- Avoid adding any other high-potassium or high-phosphorus ingredients to the salad.

- This makes a refreshing and nutrient-dense salad for someone with stage 3 chronic kidney disease.

19. Baked cod with a side of steamed broccoli

Ingredients:
- 4 oz cod fillet
- 1 tsp olive oil
- 1 tsp lemon juice
- Salt and pepper to taste (use very little salt)
- 1 cup broccoli florets

Instructions:
1. Preheat your oven to 400°F (200°C).

2. Place the cod fillet in a baking dish and drizzle with the olive oil and lemon juice. Season with a small amount of salt and pepper.

3. Bake the cod for 12-15 minutes, or until it flakes easily with a fork.

4. While the cod is baking, steam the broccoli florets until tender-crisp, about 5-7 minutes.
5. Serve the baked cod alongside the steamed broccoli.

Tips:
- Cod is a lean, low-phosphorus fish that is a good protein source.

- Broccoli is a low-potassium vegetable that provides fiber, vitamins, and minerals.

- Use just a small amount of salt, as sodium intake should be limited with stage 3 chronic kidney disease.

- Lemon juice adds flavor without the need for additional salt.

- Avoid adding any high-potassium or high-phosphorus sauces, seasonings, or toppings to the cod or broccoli.

- This makes a simple, nutrient-dense, and kidney-friendly meal.

This baked cod with steamed broccoli provides a balanced and flavorful option for someone with stage 3 chronic kidney disease. The combination of a lean protein source and a low-potassium vegetable makes it a great choice for managing kidney health.

20. Chicken and vegetable quinoa bowl

Ingredients:
- 1/2 cup cooked quinoa
- 4 oz grilled or baked chicken breast, diced
- 1/2 cup diced bell peppers
- 1/2 cup diced zucchini
- 1/4 cup diced onion
- 2 tbsp low-sodium soy sauce or tamari
- 1 tsp olive oil
- Salt and pepper to taste (use very little salt)

Instructions:
1. Cook the quinoa according to package instructions. Set aside.

2. In a large skillet or wok, heat the olive oil over medium-high heat.

3. Add the diced bell peppers, zucchini, and onion. Sauté for 5-7 minutes, until the vegetables are tender-crisp.

4. Add the diced chicken and low-sodium soy sauce or tamari. Stir to combine and heat through.

5. Scoop the chicken and vegetable mixture into a bowl and top with the cooked quinoa.

6. Season with a small amount of salt and pepper to taste.

Tips:
- Quinoa is a low-potassium, low-phosphorus grain that provides fiber and protein.

- Grilled or baked chicken breast is a lean protein source that is low in phosphorus.

- Choose a variety of low-potassium vegetables like bell peppers, zucchini, and onions.

- Use low-sodium soy sauce or tamari to keep the sodium content in check.

- Avoid adding any other high-potassium or high-phosphorus ingredients.

- This makes a complete, nutrient-dense meal that is kidney-friendly.

This chicken and vegetable quinoa bowl provides a balanced and flavorful option for someone with stage 3 chronic kidney disease. The combination of a whole grain, lean protein, and low-potassium vegetables makes it a great choice for managing kidney health.

21. Grilled salmon with a side of asparagus

Ingredients:
- 4 oz salmon fillet
- 1 tsp olive oil
- 1 tbsp lemon juice
- Salt and pepper to taste (use very little salt)
- 1 cup asparagus spears, trimmed

Instructions:
1. Preheat your grill or grill pan to medium-high heat.

2. Brush the salmon fillet with the olive oil and drizzle with the lemon juice. Season with a small amount of salt and pepper.

3. Grill the salmon for 8-10 minutes, flipping halfway, until it flakes easily with a fork.

4. While the salmon is grilling, steam the asparagus spears until tender-crisp, about 5-7 minutes.

5. Serve the grilled salmon alongside the steamed asparagus.

Tips:
- Salmon is a nutrient-dense, low-phosphorus fish that provides healthy omega-3 fatty acids.

- Asparagus is a low-potassium vegetable that provides fiber, vitamins, and minerals.

- Use just a small amount of salt, as sodium intake should be limited with stage 3 chronic kidney disease.

- Lemon juice adds flavor without the need for additional salt.

- Avoid adding any high-potassium or high-phosphorus sauces, seasonings, or toppings to the salmon or asparagus.

- This makes a simple, balanced, and kidney-friendly meal.

This grilled salmon with a side of asparagus provides a nutrient-dense and flavorful option for someone with stage 3 chronic kidney disease. The combination of a lean protein source and a low-potassium vegetable makes it a great choice for managing kidney health.

22. Beef stir-fry with bell peppers and broccoli

Ingredients:
- 4 oz lean beef, thinly sliced
- 1 tbsp low-sodium soy sauce or tamari
- 1 tsp sesame oil
- 1 cup broccoli florets
- 1/2 cup diced bell peppers
- 1/4 cup diced onion
- 1 clove garlic, minced
- 1 tsp cornstarch
- 2 tbsp water
- Salt and pepper to taste (use very little salt)

Instructions:
1. In a small bowl, combine the sliced beef, low-sodium soy sauce or tamari, and sesame oil. Set aside.

2. In a large skillet or wok, stir-fry the broccoli florets, diced bell peppers, onion, and garlic over medium-high heat for 5-7 minutes, until the vegetables are tender-crisp.

3. Add the marinated beef to the skillet and continue to stir-fry for 3-5 minutes, until the beef is cooked through.

4. In a small bowl, mix the cornstarch and water to create a slurry. Slowly pour the slurry into the skillet, stirring constantly, to thicken the sauce. Season with a small amount of salt and pepper to taste.

Tips:
- Choose a lean cut of beef to keep the phosphorus content low.

- Use low-sodium soy sauce or tamari to limit the sodium intake.

- Broccoli and bell peppers are low-potassium vegetables that add nutrients and flavor.

- The cornstarch slurry helps create a light sauce without the need for high-sodium or high-phosphorus ingredients.

- Serve the beef stir-fry over a small portion of cooked quinoa or brown rice for a complete meal.

- Avoid adding any other high-potassium or high-phosphorus ingredients.

This beef stir-fry with bell peppers and broccoli provides a nutrient-dense and kidney-friendly option for someone with stage 3 chronic kidney disease.

23. Baked chicken with rosemary and thyme

Ingredients:
- 4 oz boneless, skinless chicken breast
- 1 tsp olive oil
- 1 tsp fresh rosemary, chopped
- 1 tsp fresh thyme, chopped
- Salt and pepper to taste (use very little salt)

Instructions:
1. Preheat your oven to 400°F (200°C).

2. Place the chicken breast in a baking dish and drizzle with the olive oil, making sure to coat the chicken evenly.

3. Sprinkle the chopped rosemary and thyme over the chicken.

4. Season with a small amount of salt and pepper to taste.

5. Bake the chicken for 20-25 minutes, or until it reaches an internal temperature of 165°F (74°C). Allow the chicken to rest for a few minutes before serving.

Tips:
- Boneless, skinless chicken breast is a lean protein source that is low in phosphorus.

- Rosemary and thyme are flavorful herbs that add taste without the need for additional salt.

- Use just a small amount of salt, as sodium intake should be limited with stage 3 chronic kidney disease.

- Serve the baked chicken with a side of steamed low-potassium vegetables, such as broccoli or asparagus.

- Avoid adding any high-potassium or high-phosphorus sauces, seasonings, or toppings to the chicken.

This baked chicken with rosemary and thyme provides a simple, nutrient-dense, and kidney-friendly main dish option for someone with stage 3 chronic kidney disease. The combination of a lean protein source and flavorful herbs makes it a great choice for managing kidney health.

24. Spaghetti squash with marinara sauce

Ingredients:
- 1 medium spaghetti squash
- 1 cup low-sodium marinara sauce
- 1 tbsp grated Parmesan cheese (optional)
- Salt and pepper to taste (use very little salt)

Instructions:
1. Preheat your oven to 400°F (200°C).

2. Cut the spaghetti squash in half lengthwise and scoop out the seeds.

3. Place the squash halves cut-side down on a baking sheet lined with parchment paper.

4. Bake the squash for 30-40 minutes, or until it's tender and easily shreds with a fork.

5. Remove the squash from the oven and let it cool slightly.

6. Use a fork to shred the squash flesh into spaghetti-like strands.

7. In a saucepan, heat the low-sodium marinara sauce over medium heat.

8. Serve the spaghetti squash strands topped with the warm marinara sauce.

9. If desired, sprinkle a small amount of grated Parmesan cheese on top. Season with a small amount of salt and pepper to taste.

Tips:
- Spaghetti squash is a low-potassium, low-phosphorus vegetable that can be used as a pasta substitute.

- Choose a low-sodium marinara sauce to keep the sodium content in check.

- Parmesan cheese is a low-phosphorus cheese that can add flavor, but use it sparingly.

- Avoid adding any other high-potassium or high-phosphorus toppings or ingredients.

- Serve this dish with a side salad of mixed greens for a complete, kidney-friendly meal.

This spaghetti squash with marinara sauce provides a nutrient-dense and low-potassium alternative to traditional pasta dishes, making it a great option for someone with stage 3 chronic kidney disease.

25. Herb-roasted pork tenderloin

Ingredients:
- 1 lb pork tenderloin
- 1 tbsp olive oil
- 1 tsp dried rosemary
- 1 tsp dried thyme
- 1/2 tsp garlic powder
- Salt and pepper to taste (use very little salt)

Instructions:
1. Preheat your oven to 400°F (200°C).

2. In a small bowl, mix together the olive oil, dried rosemary, dried thyme, and garlic powder.

3. Rub the herb mixture all over the pork tenderloin, making sure to coat it evenly.

4. Season the pork with a small amount of salt and pepper.

5. Place the pork tenderloin in a baking dish or on a rimmed baking sheet.

6. Roast the pork in the preheated oven for 20-25 minutes, or until it reaches an internal temperature of 145°F (63°C). Allow the pork to rest for 5-10 minutes before slicing and serving.

Tips:
- Pork tenderloin is a lean protein source that is low in phosphorus.

- The herbs and spices add flavor without the need for additional salt.

- Use just a small amount of salt, as sodium intake should be limited with stage 3 chronic kidney disease.

- Serve the herb-roasted pork tenderloin with a side of steamed low-potassium vegetables, such as broccoli or green beans.

- Avoid adding any high-potassium or high-phosphorus sauces, gravies, or toppings to the pork.

This herb-roasted pork tenderloin provides a simple, flavorful, and kidney-friendly main dish option for someone with stage 3 chronic kidney disease. The combination of a lean protein source and aromatic herbs makes it a nutritious and satisfying choice.

26. Vegetable and tofu stir-fry

Ingredients:
- 4 oz firm or extra-firm tofu, cubed
- 1 tbsp low-sodium soy sauce or tamari
- 1 tsp sesame oil
- 1 cup mixed vegetables (such as broccoli, bell peppers, and snow peas)
- 1/4 cup diced onion
- 1 clove garlic, minced
- 1 tsp cornstarch
- 2 tbsp water
- Salt and pepper to taste (use very little salt)

Instructions:
1. In a small bowl, combine the cubed tofu, low-sodium soy sauce or tamari, and sesame oil. Set aside.

2. In a large skillet or wok, stir-fry the mixed vegetables and diced onion over medium-high heat for 5-7 minutes, until the vegetables are tender-crisp.

3. Add the marinated tofu and minced garlic to the skillet. Continue to stir-fry for 3-5 minutes, until the tofu is heated through.

4. In a small bowl, mix the cornstarch and water to create a slurry. Slowly pour the slurry into the skillet, stirring constantly, to thicken the sauce. Season with a small amount of salt and pepper to taste.

Tips:
- Firm or extra-firm tofu is a good source of plant-based protein that is low in phosphorus.

- Use low-sodium soy sauce or tamari to limit the sodium intake.

- Choose a variety of low-potassium vegetables, such as broccoli, bell peppers, and snow peas.

- The cornstarch slurry helps create a light sauce without the need for high-sodium or high-phosphorus ingredients.

- Avoid adding any other high-potassium or high-phosphorus ingredients to the stir-fry.

- Serve the vegetable and tofu stir-fry over a small portion of cooked quinoa or brown rice for a complete meal

27. Grilled shrimp with a side of green beans

Ingredients:
- 6 oz raw shrimp, peeled and deveined
- 1 tbsp olive oil
- 1 tsp lemon juice
- 1 tsp dried oregano
- Salt and pepper to taste (use very little salt)
- 1 cup fresh green beans, trimmed

Instructions:
1. Preheat your grill or grill pan to medium-high heat.

2. In a small bowl, combine the shrimp, olive oil, lemon juice, and dried oregano. Toss to coat the shrimp evenly.

3. Thread the marinated shrimp onto skewers, if desired.

4. Grill the shrimp for 2-3 minutes per side, or until they are opaque and cooked through.

5. While the shrimp are grilling, steam the green beans until tender-crisp, about 5-7 minutes.

6. Serve the grilled shrimp alongside the steamed green beans. Season the shrimp and green beans with a small amount of salt and pepper to taste.

Tips:
- Shrimp is a low-phosphorus protein source that is also low in potassium.

- Green beans are a low-potassium vegetable that provides fiber, vitamins, and minerals.

- Use just a small amount of salt, as sodium intake should be limited with stage 3 chronic kidney disease.

- Lemon juice and dried oregano add flavor without the need for additional salt.

- Avoid adding any high-potassium or high-phosphorus sauces, seasonings, or toppings to the shrimp or green beans. This makes a simple, balanced, and kidney-friendly meal.

This grilled shrimp with a side of green beans provides a nutrient-dense and flavorful option for someone with stage 3 chronic kidney disease. The combination of a lean protein source and a low-potassium vegetable makes it a great choice for managing kidney health.

28. Stuffed bell peppers with ground turkey and quinoa

Ingredients:
- 2 medium bell peppers, halved and seeded
- 4 oz ground turkey
- 1/2 cup cooked quinoa
- 1/4 cup diced onion
- 1 clove garlic, minced
- 1 tbsp low-sodium tomato sauce
- 1 tsp dried oregano
- Salt and pepper to taste (use very little salt)

Instructions:
1. Preheat your oven to 375°F (190°C).

2. In a skillet over medium heat, cook the ground turkey, diced onion, and minced garlic until the turkey is browned and the vegetables are softened, about 5-7 minutes.

3. Stir in the cooked quinoa, low-sodium tomato sauce, and dried oregano. Season with a small amount of salt and pepper to taste.

4. Spoon the turkey and quinoa mixture into the hollowed-out bell pepper halves, packing it in gently.

5. Place the stuffed bell pepper halves in a baking dish and cover with foil.

6. Bake for 20-25 minutes, or until the peppers are tender. Remove the foil and bake for an additional 5 minutes to lightly brown the tops.

Tips:
- Bell peppers are a low-potassium vegetable that provides a nutrient-dense vessel for the filling.

- Ground turkey is a lean protein source that is low in phosphorus.

- Quinoa is a low-potassium, low-phosphorus grain that adds fiber and nutrients to the filling.

- Use a small amount of low-sodium tomato sauce to add flavor without excessive sodium.

- Avoid adding any high-potassium or high-phosphorus ingredients to the stuffing. Serve the stuffed bell peppers as a main dish or alongside a small salad of mixed greens

29. Baked tilapia with lemon and dill

Ingredients:
- 4 oz tilapia fillet
- 1 tbsp lemon juice
- 1 tsp dried dill
- 1 tsp olive oil
- Salt and pepper to taste (use very little salt)

Instructions:
1. Preheat your oven to 400°F (200°C).

2. Place the tilapia fillet in a baking dish and drizzle with the lemon juice and olive oil, making sure to coat the fish evenly.

3. Sprinkle the dried dill over the top of the fish.

4. Season with a small amount of salt and pepper to taste.

5. Bake the tilapia for 12-15 minutes, or until it flakes easily with a fork.

Tips:
- Tilapia is a lean, low-phosphorus fish that is a good protein source.

- Lemon juice and dried dill add flavor without the need for additional salt.

- Use just a small amount of salt, as sodium intake should be limited with stage 3 chronic kidney disease.

- Serve the baked tilapia with a side of steamed low-potassium vegetables, such as broccoli or asparagus.

- Avoid adding any high-potassium or high-phosphorus sauces, seasonings, or toppings to the fish.

This baked tilapia with lemon and dill provides a simple, nutrient-dense, and kidney-friendly main dish option for someone with stage 3 chronic kidney disease. The combination of a lean protein source and flavorful herbs makes it a great choice for managing kidney health.

30. Eggplant parmesan (using low-sodium tomato sauce)

Ingredients:
- 1 medium eggplant, sliced into 1/4-inch thick rounds
- 1 cup low-sodium tomato sauce
- 1/2 cup shredded low-fat, low-sodium mozzarella cheese
- 2 tbsp grated Parmesan cheese
- 1 tbsp olive oil
- 1 tsp dried oregano
- Salt and pepper to taste (use very little salt)

Instructions:
1. Preheat your oven to 375°F (190°C).

2. Brush the eggplant slices lightly with the olive oil on both sides.

3. Arrange the eggplant slices in a single layer on a baking sheet.

4. Bake the eggplant for 15-20 minutes, flipping halfway, until tender and lightly browned.

5. In a baking dish, spread a thin layer of the low-sodium tomato sauce on the bottom.

6. Arrange the baked eggplant slices in a single layer on top of the sauce.

7. Top the eggplant with the shredded low-fat, low-sodium mozzarella cheese and grated Parmesan cheese. Sprinkle the dried oregano over the top.

8. Bake the eggplant parmesan for 20-25 minutes, or until the cheese is melted and bubbly. Season with a small amount of salt and pepper to taste.

Tips:
- Eggplant is a low-potassium vegetable that provides a good base for this dish.
- Use a low-sodium tomato sauce to keep the sodium content in check.
- Choose low-fat, low-sodium mozzarella cheese to limit the phosphorus and sodium.
- Parmesan cheese is a low-phosphorus cheese that can add flavor, but use it sparingly.
- Avoid adding any other high-potassium or high-phosphorus ingredients.
- Serve the eggplant parmesan with a side salad of mixed greens for a complete, kidney-friendly meal.

This eggplant parmesan with low-sodium tomato sauce provides a nutrient-dense and flavorful option for someone with stage 3 chronic kidney disease.

31. Chickpea and vegetable curry

Ingredients:
- 1 cup cooked chickpeas (garbanzo beans), rinsed and drained
- 1 cup diced bell peppers
- 1 cup diced zucchini
- 1/2 cup diced onion
- 2 cloves garlic, minced
- 1 tsp curry powder
- 1 tsp ground cumin
- 1 cup low-sodium vegetable broth
- 1 tbsp low-fat, low-sodium coconut milk (optional)
- Salt and pepper to taste (use very little salt)

Instructions:
1. In a large skillet or saucepan, sauté the diced bell peppers, zucchini, onion, and garlic over medium heat for 5-7 minutes, until the vegetables are tender.

2. Add the cooked chickpeas, curry powder, and ground cumin to the skillet. Stir to combine.

3. Pour in the low-sodium vegetable broth and bring the mixture to a simmer.

4. Reduce the heat and let the curry simmer for 10-15 minutes, allowing the flavors to meld.

5. If desired, stir in the low-fat, low-sodium coconut milk to add a creamy texture.

6. Season with a small amount of salt and pepper to taste.

Tips:
- Chickpeas are a good source of plant-based protein that is low in phosphorus.
- Bell peppers and zucchini are low-potassium vegetables that add nutrients and flavor to the curry.
- Use a low-sodium vegetable broth to keep the sodium content in check.
- The small amount of low-fat, low-sodium coconut milk can add creaminess, but it's optional.
- Avoid adding any other high-potassium or high-phosphorus ingredients to the curry.
- Serve the chickpea and vegetable curry over a small portion of cooked quinoa or brown rice for a complete meal.

This chickpea and vegetable curry provides a flavorful, nutrient-dense, and kidney-friendly option for someone with stage 3 chronic kidney disease.

32. Low-sodium meatloaf with mashed cauliflower

Ingredients:
Meatloaf:
- 1 lb ground turkey or lean ground beef
- 1/2 cup whole grain breadcrumbs
- 1/4 cup diced onion
- 1 clove garlic, minced
- 1 tbsp low-sodium ketchup
- 1 tsp dried oregano
- Salt and pepper to taste (use very little salt)

Mashed Cauliflower:
- 1 head of cauliflower, cut into florets
- 2 tbsp low-fat, low-sodium milk
- 1 tbsp grated Parmesan cheese (optional)
- Salt and pepper to taste (use very little salt)

Instructions:
Meatloaf:
1. Preheat your oven to 375°F (190°C).
2. In a large bowl, combine the ground turkey or beef, breadcrumbs, diced onion, minced garlic, low-sodium ketchup, and dried oregano. Mix well.
3. Season with a small amount of salt and pepper to taste. Shape the mixture into a loaf and place it in a baking dish.
4. Bake the meatloaf for 45-55 minutes, or until it reaches an internal temperature of 165°F (74°C).

Mashed Cauliflower:
1. In a large pot, bring water to a boil. Add the cauliflower florets and cook until tender, about 10-12 minutes.
2. Drain the cauliflower and return it to the pot.
3. Add the low-fat, low-sodium milk and mash the cauliflower until smooth.
4. Stir in the grated Parmesan cheese (if using) and season with a small amount of salt and pepper to taste.

Tips:
- Ground turkey or lean ground beef are low-phosphorus protein sources.
- Whole grain breadcrumbs provide fiber without adding excessive sodium.
- Cauliflower is a low-potassium vegetable that makes a great substitute for mashed potatoes.
- Use a small amount of low-fat, low-sodium milk and Parmesan cheese to keep the phosphorus and sodium content in check.
- Avoid adding any other high-potassium or high-phosphorus ingredients to the meatloaf or mashed cauliflower.

This low-sodium meatloaf with mashed cauliflower provides a balanced and kidney-friendly meal option for someone with stage 3 chronic kidney disease.

33. Baked chicken with a side of brown rice

Ingredients:
- 4 (6oz) boneless, skinless chicken breasts
- 2 tablespoons olive oil
- 1 teaspoon dried thyme
- 1/2 teaspoon paprika
- 1/4 teaspoon black pepper
- 1/4 teaspoon garlic powder
- Juice of 1 lemon

Instructions:
1. Preheat oven to 375°F (190°C).

2. Brush the chicken breasts with olive oil on both sides.

3. In a small bowl, mix together the thyme, paprika, black pepper, and garlic powder.

4. Sprinkle the seasoning mix evenly over both sides of the chicken breasts.

5. Place the chicken in a baking dish and pour the lemon juice over the top.

6. Bake for 25-30 minutes, or until the chicken is cooked through (internal temp of 165°F/74°C).

Brown Rice
Ingredients:
- 1 cup brown rice
- 2 cups water or low-sodium chicken broth

Instructions:
1. Rinse the brown rice in a mesh strainer.
2. In a saucepan, bring the water or broth to a boil.
3. Add the rinsed rice, stir, and return to a boil.
4. Reduce heat to low, cover, and simmer for 40-45 minutes, until rice is tender.
5. Remove from heat and let stand, covered, for 5 minutes. Fluff with a fork before serving.

This baked chicken dish is low in sodium, phosphorus, and potassium, making it suitable for those with chronic kidney disease stage 3. The brown rice provides fiber and nutrients while being relatively low in potassium compared to other grains.

34. Zucchini noodles with pesto sauce

Ingredients:
For the zucchini noodles:
- 4 medium zucchini
- 1 tbsp olive oil
- 1 clove garlic, minced
- Salt and pepper to taste

For the pesto sauce:
- 2 cups fresh basil leaves
- 1/4 cup pine nuts (or walnuts)
- 2 cloves garlic
- 1/2 cup olive oil
- 1/4 cup grated Parmesan cheese
- Salt and pepper to taste

Instructions:
1. Make the zucchini noodles:
- Use a spiralizer or julienne peeler to cut the zucchini into noodle-like strips.

- Heat olive oil in a large skillet over medium heat.

- Add the minced garlic and sauté for 30 seconds.

- Add the zucchini noodles and season with salt and pepper. Sauté for 2-3 minutes until slightly softened but still crisp. Remove from heat and set aside.

2. Make the pesto sauce:
- In a food processor, combine the basil leaves, pine nuts (or walnuts), garlic, and olive oil. Process until well combined and a coarse paste forms.

- Transfer the pesto to a bowl and stir in the grated Parmesan cheese. Season with salt and pepper to taste.

3. Combine the zucchini noodles and pesto sauce: Add the zucchini noodles to the pesto sauce and toss gently to coat.

4. Serve and enjoy!

Notes:
- This recipe is low in potassium, phosphorus, and sodium, making it suitable for those with chronic kidney disease stage 3.
- The zucchini noodles provide a low-potassium alternative to regular pasta.
- The pesto sauce is made with a moderate amount of olive oil and Parmesan cheese, which are reasonable for a kidney disease diet in moderation.
- You can adjust the amount of Parmesan cheese or omit it if needed to further reduce the phosphorus content.

35. Lentil and vegetable stew

Ingredients:
- 1 cup dried green or brown lentils, rinsed
- 4 cups low-sodium vegetable broth or water
- 1 tablespoon olive oil
- 1 onion, diced
- 2 carrots, diced
- 2 stalks celery, diced
- 2 cloves garlic, minced
- 1 teaspoon dried thyme
- 1/2 teaspoon dried rosemary
- 1/4 teaspoon black pepper
- 2 cups diced zucchini
- 1 cup diced bell pepper (any color)
- 2 tablespoons lemon juice
- Salt to taste (if needed)

Instructions:
1. In a large pot, combine the lentils and vegetable broth or water. Bring to a boil, then reduce heat to low, cover, and simmer for 20 minutes.

2. In a separate skillet, heat the olive oil over medium heat. Add the onion, carrots, and celery. Sauté for 5 minutes, until slightly softened.

3. Add the garlic, thyme, rosemary, and black pepper to the skillet. Sauté for 1 minute more.

4. Transfer the sautéed vegetable mixture to the pot with the lentils and broth. Add the diced zucchini and bell pepper.

5. Bring the stew to a simmer and cook for 15-20 minutes, until lentils and vegetables are tender.

6. Stir in the lemon juice and season with salt to taste, if needed. Serve hot, garnished with fresh parsley or cilantro if desired.

Notes:
- This stew is high in fiber, low in potassium, phosphorus, and sodium, making it suitable for those with chronic kidney disease stage 3.

- Lentils are an excellent source of plant-based protein and are low in potassium.

- The vegetables in the stew provide essential vitamins and minerals while being low in potassium and phosphorus.

- You can adjust the quantities of vegetables according to your preference or dietary needs.

- If you need to further reduce the potassium content, you can omit or reduce the bell pepper.

36. Grilled chicken with a side of quinoa salad

Ingredients:
- 4 (6 oz) boneless, skinless chicken breasts
- 2 tablespoons olive oil
- 1 teaspoon dried oregano
- 1/2 teaspoon paprika
- 1/4 teaspoon black pepper
- Juice of 1 lemon

Instructions:
1. Pound the chicken breasts to an even thickness.
2. In a shallow dish, mix together the olive oil, oregano, paprika, black pepper, and lemon juice.
3. Add the chicken breasts to the marinade and turn to coat both sides. Cover and marinate for 30 minutes to 1 hour in the refrigerator.
4. Preheat an outdoor grill or grill pan to medium-high heat.
5. Grill the chicken for 5-7 minutes per side, or until cooked through (internal temperature of 165°F/74°C).

Quinoa Salad
Ingredients:
- 1 cup quinoa, rinsed
- 2 cups low-sodium vegetable broth or water
- 1/2 cucumber, diced
- 1 tomato, diced
- 1/4 cup diced red onion
- 2 tablespoons chopped fresh parsley
- 2 tablespoons lemon juice
- 2 tablespoons olive oil
- Salt and pepper to taste

Instructions:
1. In a saucepan, bring the vegetable broth or water to a boil. Add the rinsed quinoa, reduce heat to low, cover, and simmer for 15-20 minutes, until quinoa is cooked and liquid is absorbed.
2. Transfer the cooked quinoa to a large bowl and let it cool slightly.
3. Add the diced cucumber, tomato, red onion, and chopped parsley to the quinoa.
4. Drizzle with lemon juice and olive oil, and season with salt and pepper to taste.
5. Toss gently to combine all the ingredients.

Notes:
- This meal is low in potassium, phosphorus, and sodium, making it suitable for those with chronic kidney disease stage 3.
- The grilled chicken provides a lean source of protein.
- The quinoa salad is a nutrient-dense side dish that is low in potassium and phosphorus, and high in fiber.

37. Pork chops with apple chutney

Ingredients:
- 4 (6 oz) boneless pork chops
- 1 tbsp olive oil
- 1 tsp dried thyme
- 1/2 tsp paprika
- 1/4 tsp black pepper
- 1/4 tsp garlic powder
- Salt to taste (if needed)

Instructions:

1. Pat the pork chops dry and season both sides with thyme, paprika, black pepper, and garlic powder.

2. Heat olive oil in a large skillet over medium-high heat.

3. Add the seasoned pork chops and cook for 4-5 minutes per side, or until internal temperature reaches 145°F (63°C). Transfer pork chops to a plate and tent with foil to keep warm.

Apple Chutney

Ingredients:
- 1 tsp ground cinnamon
- 1/4 tsp ground ginger
- 1/4 tsp ground allspice
- 2 Granny Smith apples, peeled, cored, and diced
- 1/2 cup water
- 2 tbsp white wine vinegar
- 2 tbsp brown sugar

Instructions:

1. In a saucepan, combine the diced apples, water, vinegar, brown sugar, cinnamon, ginger, and allspice.

2. Bring the mixture to a boil, then reduce heat and simmer for 15-20 minutes, or until the apples are tender and the chutney thickens.

3. Mash the mixture slightly with a fork or potato masher to achieve a chunky texture.

Notes:
- This meal is low in potassium, phosphorus, and sodium, making it suitable for those with chronic kidney disease stage 3.
- Pork chops are a good source of protein and low in potassium and phosphorus.
- The apple chutney is a flavorful condiment that provides a sweet and tangy accompaniment to the pork chops.
- If needed, you can adjust the amount of brown sugar in the chutney to reduce the potassium content further.
- Serve with a side of steamed low-potassium vegetables or a small portion of rice or quinoa for a complete meal.

38. Vegetable lasagna (using whole wheat noodles)

Ingredients:
For the vegetable filling:
- 1 tbsp olive oil
- 1 onion, diced
- 3 cloves garlic, minced
- 2 cups sliced mushrooms
- 2 zucchini, diced
- 1 red bell pepper, diced
- 1 (15 oz) can low-sodium tomato sauce
- 1 tsp dried basil
- 1 tsp dried oregano
- Salt and pepper to taste

For the cheese sauce:
- 2 tbsp butter
- 2 tbsp all-purpose flour
- 2 cups low-fat milk
- 1/2 cup grated Parmesan cheese
- Salt and pepper to taste

Other ingredients:
- 9 whole wheat lasagna noodles
- 1 cup low-fat ricotta cheese
- 1 cup shredded low-fat mozzarella cheese

Instructions:

1. Preheat oven to 375°F (190°C).

2. Make the vegetable filling: Heat olive oil in a large skillet over medium heat. Sauté the onion and garlic until fragrant, about 2 minutes. Add the mushrooms, zucchini, and bell pepper. Cook for 5-7 minutes until vegetables are tender. Stir in the tomato sauce, basil, oregano, and season with salt and pepper to taste.

3. Make the cheese sauce: In a saucepan, melt the butter over medium heat. Whisk in the flour and cook for 2 minutes. Gradually whisk in the milk and cook until thickened, about 5 minutes. Remove from heat and stir in the Parmesan cheese. Season with salt and pepper to taste.

4. Cook the lasagna noodles according to package instructions until al dente. Drain and rinse with cold water.

5. In a 9x13 inch baking dish, spread a thin layer of the cheese sauce. Layer with 3 lasagna noodles, half of the vegetable filling, 1/3 of the remaining cheese sauce, and 1/2 of the ricotta cheese. Repeat with another layer of noodles, remaining vegetable filling, 1/3 of the cheese sauce, and the remaining ricotta cheese. Top with the remaining 3 lasagna noodles and the remaining cheese sauce.

6. Cover with aluminum foil and bake for 25 minutes. Remove the foil, sprinkle with the shredded mozzarella cheese, and bake for an additional 10-15 minutes, or until the cheese is melted and bubbly. Let the lasagna rest for 10 minutes before slicing and serving.

39. Turkey meatballs with a side of green beans

Ingredients:
- 1 lb lean ground turkey
- 1/2 cup low-sodium breadcrumbs
- 1 egg
- 1/4 cup finely chopped onion
- 1 minced garlic clove
- 1 tbsp chopped parsley (optional)
- 1/4 tsp black pepper
- 1/4 tsp dried oregano
- 1 tbsp olive oil

Instructions:
1. Mix turkey, breadcrumbs, egg, onion, garlic, parsley, pepper, and oregano.

2. Form into 1-inch meatballs.

3. Heat olive oil in a skillet over medium heat.

4. Cook meatballs for 10-12 minutes, turning occasionally, until browned and cooked through. Drain on a paper towel-lined plate.

Green Beans
Ingredients:
- 1 lb fresh green beans, trimmed
- 1 tbsp olive oil
- 1 minced garlic clove
- 1/4 tsp black pepper
- 1 tbsp lemon juice

Instructions:
1. Blanch green beans in boiling water for 3-4 minutes.

2. Drain and cool in ice water. Drain again.

3. Heat olive oil in a skillet over medium heat.

4. Sauté garlic for 1 minute.

5. Add green beans and sauté for 3-4 minutes.

6. Season with pepper and drizzle with lemon juice.

Enjoy your meal! Consult your healthcare provider to ensure these recipes fit your dietary needs.

40. Grilled vegetable kebabs

Ingredients:
- 1 red bell pepper, cut into 1-inch pieces
- 1 yellow bell pepper, cut into 1-inch pieces
- 1 zucchini, cut into 1/2-inch rounds
- 1 yellow squash, cut into 1/2-inch rounds
- 8 cherry tomatoes
- 1 small red onion, cut into wedges
- 1/4 cup olive oil
- 2 tbsp lemon juice
- 1 tsp dried oregano
- 1/4 tsp black pepper
- 2 cloves garlic, minced

Instructions:
1. Preheat grill to medium-high heat.

2. In a small bowl, whisk together olive oil, lemon juice, oregano, black pepper, and garlic.

3. Thread the vegetables onto skewers, alternating between different types.

4. Brush the vegetable skewers with the olive oil mixture.

5. Grill the kebabs for 10-12 minutes, turning occasionally, until vegetables are tender and slightly charred. Serve immediately.

Nutritional Considerations:
- Low Sodium: These kebabs are naturally low in sodium.

- Potassium and Phosphorus: The selected vegetables are relatively low in potassium and phosphorus, suitable for a CKD-friendly diet.

- Hydration: Grilling vegetables helps retain their moisture, making them more enjoyable and kidney-friendly.

Enjoy your kidney-friendly grilled vegetable kebabs! Always consult your healthcare provider or a registered dietitian to ensure these recipes fit your specific dietary needs.

41. Apple slices with almond butter

Ingredients:
- 1 medium apple, sliced
- 2 tablespoons almond butter (unsweetened, no added salt)

Instructions:
1. Wash and slice the apple into thin wedges.

2. Spread almond butter on each apple slice or serve it on the side for dipping.

Nutritional Considerations:

- Low Sodium: Almond butter and apples are naturally low in sodium.

- Moderate Potassium: Apples are relatively low in potassium, making them a good choice for CKD patients in moderation.

- Healthy Fats: Almond butter provides healthy fats and protein, which are beneficial in controlled amounts for kidney health.

Enjoy this simple, kidney-friendly snack! Always consult with your healthcare provider or a registered dietitian to ensure these recipes align with your dietary needs.

42. Carrot sticks with hummus

Ingredients:
- 4 medium carrots, peeled and cut into sticks
- 1/2 cup hummus (low sodium, store-bought or homemade)

Instructions:
1. Wash, peel, and cut the carrots into sticks.

2. Serve the carrot sticks with hummus on the side for dipping.

Homemade Low-Sodium Hummus Recipe

Ingredients:
- 1 can (15 oz) chickpeas, drained and rinsed
- 2 tbsp tahini
- 2 tbsp lemon juice
- 1 clove garlic, minced
- 1/4 cup water (adjust for desired consistency)
- 1 tbsp olive oil
- 1/4 tsp cumin
- 1/4 tsp black pepper

Instructions:
1. In a food processor, combine chickpeas, tahini, lemon juice, garlic, water, olive oil, cumin, and black pepper.

2. Blend until smooth, adding more water if needed to reach the desired consistency.

3. Serve immediately or refrigerate until ready to use.

Nutritional Considerations:
- Low Sodium: Using low-sodium hummus and fresh carrots keeps sodium intake in check.

- Potassium and Phosphorus: Carrots are relatively low in potassium and phosphorus, suitable for CKD patients in moderation.

- Healthy Snack: This combination provides fiber and healthy fats, making it a nutritious and kidney-friendly snack option.

Enjoy your kidney-friendly carrot sticks with hummus! Always consult your healthcare provider or a registered dietitian to ensure these recipes fit your specific dietary needs.

43. Celery sticks with cream cheese

Ingredients:
- 4 celery stalks, cut into sticks
- 1/4 cup cream cheese (low-fat, unsalted)

Instructions:
1. Wash and cut the celery stalks into sticks.

2. Spread a small amount of cream cheese on each celery stick or serve it on the side for dipping.

Nutritional Considerations:

- Low Sodium: Using unsalted cream cheese helps keep sodium levels in check.

- Potassium and Phosphorus: Celery is low in potassium and phosphorus, making it suitable for a CKD-friendly diet.

- Healthy Fats: Low-fat cream cheese provides a source of healthy fats without overloading on calories or saturated fat.

Enjoy this simple and kidney-friendly snack! Always consult your healthcare provider or a registered dietitian to ensure these recipes align with your dietary needs.

44. Unsalted mixed nuts

Ingredients:
- 1/4 cup unsalted mixed nuts (e.g., almonds, walnuts, pecans, cashews)

Instructions:
1. Measure out 1/4 cup of unsalted mixed nuts.

2. Serve as a snack or portion into small bags for convenient, kidney-friendly snacking.

Nutritional Considerations:

- Low Sodium: Choose unsalted nuts to keep sodium intake low.

- Moderate Protein: Nuts provide a moderate amount of protein, which is suitable for CKD stage 3 when consumed in controlled portions.

- Healthy Fats: Nuts are rich in healthy fats, which are beneficial for overall health but should be eaten in moderation.

- Mineral Content: Be mindful of portion sizes, as nuts contain potassium and phosphorus, which need to be managed in a CKD diet.

Enjoy your unsalted mixed nuts in moderation! Always consult with your healthcare provider or a registered dietitian to ensure these snacks fit your specific dietary needs.

45. Rice cakes with low-sodium cheese

Ingredients:
- 2 plain rice cakes
- 2 slices low-sodium cheese (such as Swiss or mozzarella)

Instructions:
1. Place the rice cakes on a plate.

2. Top each rice cake with a slice of low-sodium cheese.

3. Optionally, you can melt the cheese slightly by microwaving for 10-15 seconds or using a toaster oven.

Nutritional Considerations:

- Low Sodium: Use low-sodium cheese to keep sodium intake in check.

- Protein: The cheese provides a good source of protein, suitable for CKD patients when consumed in moderation.

- Carbohydrates: Rice cakes provide a light, low-calorie source of carbohydrates.

Enjoy this simple, kidney-friendly snack! Always consult with your healthcare provider or a registered dietitian to ensure these recipes align with your specific dietary needs.

46. Fresh fruit salad

Ingredients:
- 1 cup strawberries, hulled and sliced
- 1 cup blueberries
- 1 cup pineapple, diced
- 1 cup apple, diced
- 1 cup grapes, halved
- 1 tbsp lemon juice (optional, to prevent apple from browning)

Instructions:
1. Wash all fruits thoroughly.

2. Hull and slice the strawberries.

3. Dice the pineapple and apple into bite-sized pieces.

4. Halve the grapes.

5. In a large bowl, combine all the fruits.

6. Optionally, drizzle with lemon juice to prevent the apple from browning and toss gently to mix.

Nutritional Considerations:

- Low Sodium: Fresh fruits are naturally low in sodium.

- Moderate Potassium: Choose fruits that are lower in potassium (e.g., berries, apples, grapes) and consume in moderation.

- Hydration: Fresh fruits have high water content, which is beneficial for hydration.

Enjoy your fresh fruit salad! Always consult with your healthcare provider or a registered dietitian to ensure these recipes fit your specific dietary needs.

47. Low-sodium popcorn

Ingredients:
- 1/4 cup popcorn kernels
- 1-2 teaspoons olive oil (optional for flavor)
- 1/4 teaspoon salt-free seasoning (optional)

Instructions:
1. Air-Popped Method:
   - Add 1/4 cup popcorn kernels to an air popper and pop according to the manufacturer's instructions.

   - If using olive oil, drizzle it over the popcorn and toss to coat evenly.

   - Sprinkle with salt-free seasoning, if desired, and toss to coat.

2. Stovetop Method:
   - Heat a large pot with a lid over medium heat and add 1-2 teaspoons of olive oil.

   - Add 1/4 cup popcorn kernels and cover the pot with the lid.

   - Shake the pot occasionally to prevent the kernels from burning.

   - Continue cooking until popping slows to a few seconds between pops, then remove from heat.

   - Sprinkle with salt-free seasoning, if desired, and toss to coat.

Nutritional Considerations:
- Low Sodium: Using no added salt and optional salt-free seasoning keeps sodium levels low.

- Whole Grains: Popcorn is a whole grain and provides fiber, which is beneficial for overall health.

- Healthy Snack: Air-popped popcorn is low in calories and a healthy snack option when not overloaded with butter or salt.

Enjoy your kidney-friendly, low-sodium popcorn! Always consult with your healthcare provider or a registered dietitian to ensure these snacks fit your specific dietary needs.

48. Bell pepper slices with guacamole

Ingredients:
- 2 bell peppers (red, yellow, or green), sliced
- 1 ripe avocado
- 1 tablespoon lime juice
- 1/4 teaspoon garlic powder
- 1/4 teaspoon onion powder
- Salt to taste (optional)
- Optional toppings: chopped tomatoes, diced onions, chopped cilantro

Instructions:
1. Wash the bell peppers, cut them in half, remove the seeds, and slice into strips.

2. Scoop the flesh of the avocado into a bowl and mash it with a fork until smooth.

3. Add lime juice, garlic powder, onion powder, and salt to the mashed avocado. Mix well.

4. Arrange the bell pepper slices on a plate and serve with the guacamole.

5. Optionally, top the guacamole with chopped tomatoes, diced onions, or chopped cilantro for added flavor and texture.

Nutritional Considerations:

- Low Sodium: Guacamole made without added salt helps control sodium intake.

- Healthy Fats: Avocado provides heart-healthy monounsaturated fats, beneficial for kidney health.

- Moderate Potassium: Bell peppers are lower in potassium compared to other fruits and vegetables, making them a suitable choice for CKD patients when consumed in moderation.

Enjoy your kidney-friendly bell pepper slices with guacamole! As always, consult with your healthcare provider or a registered dietitian for personalized dietary recommendations.

49. Cucumber slices with tzatziki

Ingredients:
- 1 medium cucumber, sliced
- 1/2 cup plain Greek yogurt (low-fat or non-fat)
- 1/4 cup grated cucumber (from the same cucumber)
- 1 clove garlic, minced
- 1 tablespoon lemon juice
- 1 tablespoon chopped fresh dill (or 1 teaspoon dried dill)
- Salt to taste (optional)
- Black pepper to taste

Instructions:
1. Wash the cucumber, slice it into thin rounds, and set aside.

2. Grate 1/4 cup of the cucumber and squeeze out excess moisture using a paper towel or clean cloth.

3. In a bowl, combine the grated cucumber, Greek yogurt, minced garlic, lemon juice, and chopped dill. Mix well.

4. Season the tzatziki with salt and black pepper to taste, if desired.

5. Arrange the cucumber slices on a serving platter and serve with the tzatziki for dipping.

Nutritional Considerations:

- Low Sodium: Using plain Greek yogurt without added salt helps control sodium intake.

- Protein: Greek yogurt provides a good source of protein, suitable for CKD patients when consumed in moderation.

- Hydration: Cucumbers have high water content, which is beneficial for hydration.

Enjoy your kidney-friendly cucumber slices with tzatziki! Always consult with your healthcare provider or a registered dietitian to ensure these recipes fit your specific dietary needs.

50. Berries with Greek yogurt

Ingredients:
- 1/2 cup mixed berries (such as strawberries, blueberries, raspberries)
- 1/2 cup plain Greek yogurt (low-fat or non-fat)
- 1 teaspoon honey or maple syrup (optional, for sweetness)
- Fresh mint leaves for garnish (optional)

Instructions:
1. Wash the berries and pat them dry with a paper towel.

2. If using strawberries, hull and slice them.

3. In a bowl, combine the Greek yogurt with honey or maple syrup if using, and mix well.

4. Spoon the Greek yogurt into a serving bowl.

5. Arrange the mixed berries on top of the Greek yogurt.

6. Garnish with fresh mint leaves if desired.

Nutritional Considerations:

- Low Sodium: Using plain Greek yogurt without added salt helps control sodium intake.

- Protein: Greek yogurt provides a good source of protein, suitable for CKD patients when consumed in moderation.

- Antioxidants and Fiber: Berries are rich in antioxidants and fiber, which are beneficial for overall health.

Enjoy your kidney-friendly berries with Greek yogurt! Always consult with your healthcare provider or a registered dietitian to ensure these recipes fit your specific dietary needs.

51. Cherry tomatoes with mozzarella

Ingredients:
- 1 cup cherry tomatoes
- 1/2 cup fresh mozzarella balls (bocconcini)
- Fresh basil leaves, torn (optional)
- Balsamic glaze for drizzling (optional)
- Salt and black pepper to taste (optional)

Instructions:
1. Wash the cherry tomatoes and pat them dry with a paper towel.

2. Drain the fresh mozzarella balls if they are stored in liquid.

3. Arrange the cherry tomatoes and mozzarella balls on a serving platter.

4. Optionally, scatter torn fresh basil leaves over the tomatoes and mozzarella.

5. Drizzle with balsamic glaze for added flavor, if desired.

6. Season with salt and black pepper to taste, if desired.

Nutritional Considerations:

- Low Sodium: Opt for fresh mozzarella and use salt sparingly to control sodium intake.

- Protein: Fresh mozzarella provides a moderate amount of protein, suitable for CKD patients when consumed in moderation.

- Antioxidants: Cherry tomatoes are rich in antioxidants and vitamins, which are beneficial for overall health.

Enjoy your kidney-friendly cherry tomatoes with mozzarella! Always consult with your healthcare provider or a registered dietitian to ensure these recipes fit your specific dietary needs.

52. Sliced pears with cottage cheese

Ingredients:
- 1 ripe pear, sliced
- 1/2 cup low-fat cottage cheese
- 1 tablespoon honey or maple syrup (optional, for sweetness)
- Ground cinnamon for sprinkling (optional)

Instructions:
1. Wash and slice the pear into thin slices.

2. Spoon the cottage cheese onto a serving plate or bowl.

3. Arrange the sliced pears alongside the cottage cheese.

4. Optionally, drizzle honey or maple syrup over the pears for sweetness.

5. Sprinkle ground cinnamon over the top, if desired.

Nutritional Considerations:

- Low Sodium: Opt for low-sodium cottage cheese to control sodium intake.

- Protein: Cottage cheese provides a good source of protein, suitable for CKD patients when consumed in moderation.

- Fiber and Vitamins: Pears are rich in fiber and vitamins, which are beneficial for overall health.

Enjoy your kidney-friendly sliced pears with cottage cheese! Always consult with your healthcare provider or a registered dietitian to ensure these recipes fit your specific dietary needs.

53. Kale chips (homemade, low sodium)

Ingredients:
- 1 bunch of kale
- 1 tablespoon olive oil
- Salt-free seasoning blend (such as garlic powder, onion powder, paprika)
- Optional: nutritional yeast for added flavor

Instructions:
1. Preheat your oven to 300°F (150°C) and line a baking sheet with parchment paper.

2. Wash the kale leaves and dry them thoroughly with a clean kitchen towel or paper towels.

3. Remove the tough stems from the kale leaves and tear the leaves into bite-sized pieces.

4. In a large bowl, drizzle the kale pieces with olive oil and toss to coat evenly.

5. Sprinkle the kale with your desired salt-free seasoning blend and optional nutritional yeast. Toss again to ensure even coating.

6. Spread the kale pieces in a single layer on the prepared baking sheet.

7. Bake in the preheated oven for about 15-20 minutes, or until the kale chips are crispy but not burnt.

8. Remove from the oven and let cool slightly before serving.

Nutritional Considerations:

- Low Sodium: Using salt-free seasoning helps control sodium intake.

- High in Fiber and Vitamins: Kale is rich in fiber, vitamins A, C, and K, which are beneficial for kidney health and overall well-being.

- Healthy Snack: Kale chips provide a crunchy and satisfying snack option that is low in calories and high in nutrients.

Enjoy your kidney-friendly homemade kale chips as a nutritious snack! Always consult with your healthcare provider or a registered dietitian to ensure these snacks fit your specific dietary needs.

54. Baked apple slices with cinnamon

Ingredients:
- 2 apples (such as Granny Smith or Honeycrisp), cored and sliced
- 1 teaspoon ground cinnamon
- 1 tablespoon honey or maple syrup (optional, for added sweetness)
- 1 tablespoon lemon juice (optional, to prevent browning)

Instructions:
1. Preheat your oven to 350°F (175°C).

2. Core the apples and slice them into thin rounds or wedges.

3. Arrange the apple slices in a single layer on a baking sheet lined with parchment paper.

4. If desired, drizzle the apple slices with lemon juice to prevent browning.

5. Sprinkle ground cinnamon evenly over the apple slices.

6. Optionally, drizzle honey or maple syrup over the apple slices for added sweetness.

7. Bake in the preheated oven for about 15-20 minutes, or until the apples are tender and slightly caramelized. Remove from the oven and let cool slightly before serving.

Nutritional Considerations:

- Low Sodium: This recipe is naturally low in sodium.

- High in Fiber and Antioxidants: Apples are rich in fiber and antioxidants, which are beneficial for kidney health.

- Moderate Potassium: While apples contain potassium, they can be included in moderation in a CKD diet.

Enjoy your kidney-friendly baked apple slices with cinnamon as a delicious and comforting dessert or snack! Always consult with your healthcare provider or a registered dietitian to ensure these recipes fit your specific dietary needs.

55. Grapes with a handful of almonds

Ingredients:
- 1 cup of grapes (preferably seedless)
- A handful of unsalted almonds

Instructions:
1. Rinse the grapes thoroughly under cold water and pat them dry with a paper towel.

2. Remove any stems or debris from the grapes.

3. Place the grapes in a serving bowl.

4. Take a handful of unsalted almonds and add them to the bowl with the grapes.

5. Gently toss the grapes and almonds together to mix them evenly.

6. Serve immediately and enjoy!

This snack provides a good balance of natural sugars from the grapes and healthy fats and protein from the almonds. Remember to consult with a healthcare professional or a registered dietitian for personalized dietary recommendations based on your individual health needs.

56. Dried apple chips

Ingredients:
- 2-3 large apples (choose a variety like Granny Smith or Fuji)
- Lemon juice (optional, for preventing browning)

Instructions:
1. Preheat your oven to 200°F (93°C) and line a baking sheet with parchment paper.

2. Wash the apples thoroughly under cold water and pat them dry with a paper towel.

3. Core the apples and slice them thinly, about 1/8 inch thick. You can use a knife or a mandoline slicer for uniform slices.

4. If desired, you can dip the apple slices in lemon juice to prevent browning. This step is optional but can help maintain the color of the apple chips.

5. Arrange the apple slices in a single layer on the prepared baking sheet, making sure they are not overlapping.

6. Place the baking sheet in the preheated oven and bake the apple slices for 1.5 to 2 hours, or until they are dried and crispy. Flip the slices halfway through the baking time to ensure even drying.

7. Once the apple chips are crispy and golden brown, remove them from the oven and let them cool completely on the baking sheet.

8. Once cooled, transfer the apple chips to an airtight container for storage. They can be kept at room temperature for several days.

Enjoy these homemade dried apple chips as a kidney-friendly snack. They provide a crunchy texture and natural sweetness without added sugars or unhealthy fats. As always, consult with a healthcare professional or a registered dietitian for personalized dietary recommendations based on your individual health needs.

57. Unsweetened applesauce

Ingredients:
- 4-5 medium-sized apples (choose a variety like Granny Smith or Fuji)
- Water
- Lemon juice (optional, for preventing browning)

Instructions:
1. Wash the apples thoroughly under cold water and pat them dry with a paper towel.

2. Core the apples and cut them into chunks. You can peel the apples if desired, but leaving the peels on can add extra fiber.

3. Place the apple chunks in a saucepan and add enough water to cover the bottom of the pan, about 1/4 inch.

4. If desired, you can add a splash of lemon juice to the apples to prevent browning.

5. Cover the saucepan with a lid and cook the apples over medium heat for 10-15 minutes, or until they are soft and tender.

6. Once the apples are cooked, remove the saucepan from the heat and let the apples cool slightly.

7. Use a potato masher or fork to mash the cooked apples until you reach your desired consistency. For smoother applesauce, you can use a blender or food processor.

8. Taste the applesauce and adjust the sweetness if necessary. If the apples are naturally sweet, you may not need to add any sweeteners. If desired, you can add a small amount of honey or cinnamon for flavor.

9. Let the applesauce cool completely before transferring it to an airtight container for storage.

10. Store the unsweetened applesauce in the refrigerator for up to one week.

Enjoy this homemade unsweetened applesauce as a kidney-friendly snack or use it as a topping for oatmeal, yogurt, or baked goods. As always, consult with a healthcare professional or a registered dietitian for personalized dietary recommendations based on your individual health needs.

58. Protein smoothie (using almond milk and low-potassium fruits)

Ingredients:
- 1 cup unsweetened almond milk (check for phosphorus additives in the ingredients)
- 1/2 cup low-potassium fruits (such as strawberries, blueberries, or peaches)
- 1/4 cup plain Greek yogurt (choose low-fat or non-fat options)
- 1 scoop of protein powder (choose a brand with low phosphorus and potassium content)
- 1 tablespoon ground flaxseed (optional, for added fiber and omega-3 fatty acids)
- Ice cubes (optional, for desired consistency)

Instructions:

1. Wash the fruits thoroughly under cold water and prepare them by removing any stems, pits, or cores.

2. In a blender, combine the unsweetened almond milk, low-potassium fruits, plain Greek yogurt, protein powder, and ground flaxseed.

3. If desired, add a few ice cubes to the blender for a colder and thicker smoothie.

4. Blend all the ingredients together until smooth and creamy. If the smoothie is too thick, you can add more almond milk to reach your desired consistency.

5. Taste the smoothie and adjust the sweetness if necessary. If desired, you can add a small amount of honey or stevia for sweetness.

6. Once blended to your liking, pour the smoothie into a glass and serve immediately.

This protein smoothie is kidney-friendly, providing a good source of protein, vitamins, and minerals without high levels of phosphorus or potassium. It's a nutritious and delicious option for individuals with stage 3 chronic kidney disease. As always, consult with a healthcare professional or a registered dietitian for personalized dietary recommendations based on your individual health needs.

59. Avocado slices with a sprinkle of lemon

Ingredients:
- 1 ripe avocado
- Fresh lemon juice

Instructions:
1. Start by selecting a ripe avocado. It should yield slightly to gentle pressure when squeezed, but not be overly mushy.

2. Wash the avocado under cold water and pat it dry with a paper towel.

3. Slice the avocado in half lengthwise and remove the pit. Use a spoon to scoop out the flesh from each half.

4. Cut the avocado halves into thin slices or cubes, depending on your preference.

5. Arrange the avocado slices on a plate or serving dish.

6. Squeeze fresh lemon juice over the avocado slices. The lemon juice not only adds flavor but also helps prevent the avocado from browning.

7. Serve the avocado slices immediately as a snack or side dish.

Enjoy the creamy texture and mild flavor of the avocado slices with a hint of tanginess from the lemon juice. This snack provides healthy fats and nutrients without excess potassium, making it suitable for individuals with chronic kidney disease. As always, consult with a healthcare professional or a registered dietitian for personalized dietary recommendations based on your individual health needs.

60. Low-sodium crackers with hummus

Ingredients:
- Low-sodium crackers (look for varieties with less than 100mg of sodium per serving)
- Hummus (store-bought or homemade)

Instructions:

1. Choose your favorite low-sodium crackers. You can opt for whole grain crackers or those made with seeds for added nutrition.

2. If you're using store-bought hummus, check the label to ensure it's low in sodium. Alternatively, you can make your own hummus using low-sodium ingredients.

3. Scoop a generous amount of hummus into a small bowl or serving dish.

4. Arrange the low-sodium crackers on a plate or serving tray.

5. Dip the crackers into the hummus and enjoy!

This snack provides a good balance of carbohydrates, protein, and healthy fats. The crackers offer fiber and carbohydrates, while the hummus provides protein and flavor. Plus, by choosing low-sodium options, you can help manage your sodium intake, which is important for kidney health. As always, consult with a healthcare professional or a registered dietitian for personalized dietary recommendations based on your individual health needs.

61. Berry sorbet

Ingredients:
- 2 cups of mixed berries (such as strawberries, blueberries, raspberries, or blackberries)
- 1/4 cup of water
- 2-3 tablespoons of honey or sugar substitute (optional, adjust to taste)
- 1 tablespoon of lemon juice (optional, for added tartness)

Instructions:
1. Wash the berries under cold water and remove any stems or debris.

2. Place the berries in a blender or food processor.

3. Add the water and optional honey or sugar substitute to the blender.

4. If using, add the lemon juice to the blender for added tartness.

5. Blend the ingredients until smooth and well combined. If the mixture is too thick, you can add a little more water to reach your desired consistency.

6. Taste the mixture and adjust the sweetness if necessary by adding more honey or sugar substitute.

7. Once the sorbet mixture is smooth and sweetened to your liking, transfer it to a shallow dish or baking pan.

8. Place the dish or pan in the freezer and let the sorbet freeze for about 2-3 hours, or until it is firm.

9. Once the sorbet is frozen, remove it from the freezer and let it sit at room temperature for a few minutes to soften slightly.

10. Use a spoon or ice cream scoop to scoop the sorbet into serving bowls or cones.

11. Garnish the berry sorbet with fresh berries or mint leaves if desired, and serve immediately.

Enjoy this homemade berry sorbet as a kidney-friendly dessert or treat. It's naturally sweetened with fruit and can be customized with your favorite berries. As always, consult with a healthcare professional or a registered dietitian for personalized dietary recommendations based on your individual health needs.

62. Rice pudding with almond milk

Ingredients:
- 1/2 cup of white rice (choose a low-phosphorus variety if available)
- 2 cups of unsweetened almond milk
- 1/4 cup of granulated sugar or sugar substitute (adjust to taste)
- 1 teaspoon of vanilla extract
- Ground cinnamon or nutmeg for garnish (optional)

Instructions:
1. Rinse the rice under cold water until the water runs clear. This helps remove excess starch.

2. In a medium saucepan, combine the rinsed rice and almond milk.

3. Bring the mixture to a gentle boil over medium heat, then reduce the heat to low and let it simmer.

4. Cook the rice, stirring occasionally, for about 20-25 minutes or until it is tender and the mixture has thickened.

5. Stir in the granulated sugar or sugar substitute and vanilla extract. Continue to cook for an additional 5 minutes, stirring occasionally, until the sugar is dissolved and the pudding is creamy.

6. Remove the saucepan from the heat and let the rice pudding cool slightly.

7. Transfer the rice pudding to serving bowls or individual containers.

8. If desired, sprinkle ground cinnamon or nutmeg on top for added flavor and garnish.

9. Serve the rice pudding warm or chilled, depending on your preference.

Enjoy this creamy and comforting rice pudding made with almond milk. It's a kidney-friendly dessert option that's lower in phosphorus compared to traditional dairy-based rice pudding recipes. As always, consult with a healthcare professional or a registered dietitian for personalized dietary recommendations based on your individual health needs.

63. Lemon sorbet

Ingredients:
- 1 cup of freshly squeezed lemon juice (about 4-6 lemons)
- 1 cup of water
- 3/4 cup of granulated sugar or sugar substitute (adjust to taste)
- Zest of 1 lemon (optional, for extra flavor)

Instructions:
1. In a small saucepan, combine the water and granulated sugar over medium heat. Stir until the sugar is completely dissolved, creating a simple syrup. This usually takes about 3-5 minutes. Remove from heat and let it cool.

2. While the syrup is cooling, juice the lemons to obtain 1 cup of freshly squeezed lemon juice. If using lemon zest, grate the zest from one lemon using a fine grater.

3. In a mixing bowl, combine the lemon juice, cooled simple syrup, and lemon zest (if using). Stir until well combined.

4. Transfer the mixture to a shallow dish or baking pan.

5. Place the dish or pan in the freezer and let the sorbet freeze for about 2-3 hours, or until it is firm.

6. Every 30 minutes during the freezing process, remove the sorbet from the freezer and stir it with a fork to break up any ice crystals and maintain a smooth texture.

7. Once the sorbet is frozen and has reached your desired consistency, remove it from the freezer.

8. Use a spoon or ice cream scoop to scoop the lemon sorbet into serving bowls or cones.

9. Garnish with fresh mint leaves or lemon slices if desired, and serve immediately.

Enjoy this homemade lemon sorbet as a kidney-friendly dessert or palate cleanser. It's light, tangy, and perfect for hot days. As always, consult with a healthcare professional or a registered dietitian for personalized dietary recommendations based on your individual health needs.

64. Gelatin dessert with fresh fruit

Ingredients:
- 1 package (3 oz) of sugar-free gelatin mix (choose a flavor of your preference)
- 1 cup of boiling water
- 1 cup of cold water
- 1 cup of diced fresh fruit (such as berries, peaches, or pineapple)
- Fresh mint leaves for garnish (optional)

Instructions:
1. In a heatproof bowl, dissolve the sugar-free gelatin mix in 1 cup of boiling water. Stir until the gelatin is completely dissolved.

2. Stir in 1 cup of cold water into the gelatin mixture.

3. Let the gelatin mixture cool for a few minutes until it reaches room temperature.

4. Meanwhile, prepare the fresh fruit by washing, peeling (if necessary), and dicing it into bite-sized pieces.

5. Once the gelatin mixture has cooled, stir in the diced fresh fruit until well combined.

6. Pour the gelatin mixture with fruit into individual serving bowls or a large serving dish.

7. Place the dish in the refrigerator and let the gelatin set for at least 2-3 hours, or until firm.

8. Once the gelatin has set, remove it from the refrigerator.

9. Garnish with fresh mint leaves if desired before serving.

Enjoy this kidney-friendly gelatin dessert with fresh fruit as a light and refreshing treat. It's low in potassium and phosphorus, making it suitable for individuals with chronic kidney disease. As always, consult with a healthcare professional or a registered dietitian for personalized dietary recommendations based on your individual health needs.

65. Coconut macaroons

Ingredients:
- 3 cups of shredded unsweetened coconut
- 3/4 cup of granulated sugar or sugar substitute (adjust to taste)
- 3 large egg whites
- 1 teaspoon of vanilla extract
- Pinch of salt

Instructions:
1. Preheat your oven to 325°F (160°C). Line a baking sheet with parchment paper or silicone baking mat.

2. In a large mixing bowl, combine the shredded unsweetened coconut and granulated sugar.

3. In a separate bowl, whisk the egg whites until they become frothy.

4. Add the frothy egg whites, vanilla extract, and a pinch of salt to the coconut mixture. Stir until well combined.

5. Using a spoon or cookie scoop, portion the coconut mixture into small mounds and place them onto the prepared baking sheet, leaving some space between each macaroon.

6. Bake the macaroons in the preheated oven for about 20-25 minutes, or until they are lightly golden brown on the outside.

7. Remove the macaroons from the oven and let them cool on the baking sheet for a few minutes.

8. Once cooled, transfer the macaroons to a wire rack to cool completely.

9. Store the coconut macaroons in an airtight container at room temperature for up to a week.

Enjoy these homemade coconut macaroons as a kidney-friendly dessert or snack. They're naturally low in sodium and phosphorus, making them suitable for individuals with chronic kidney disease. As always, consult with a healthcare professional or a registered dietitian for personalized dietary recommendations based on your individual health needs.

66. Angel food cake with strawberries

Ingredients:
- 1 prepared angel food cake (store-bought or homemade)
- 2 cups of fresh strawberries, washed, hulled, and sliced
- 1-2 tablespoons of granulated sugar or sugar substitute (optional, adjust to taste)
- Light whipped cream or whipped topping (optional, for serving)

Instructions:
1. If using store-bought angel food cake, slice it into individual servings or into slices.
   If making homemade angel food cake, follow your preferred recipe and allow it to cool completely before slicing.

2. In a mixing bowl, combine the sliced strawberries and granulated sugar or sugar substitute (if using). Stir gently to coat the strawberries in the sugar. Let the strawberries sit for about 10-15 minutes to macerate, releasing their natural juices.

3. To serve, place a slice of angel food cake on a plate or serving dish.

4. Spoon the macerated strawberries over the angel food cake slice, allowing the juices to soak into the cake.

5. Optional: Serve with a dollop of light whipped cream or whipped topping on top of the strawberries.

6. Repeat the process for each serving of angel food cake with strawberries.

7. Serve immediately and enjoy!

This dessert is light, refreshing, and perfect for summertime. The angel food cake is low in fat and provides a light, airy texture, while the fresh strawberries add natural sweetness and a burst of flavor. As always, consult with a healthcare professional or a registered dietitian for personalized dietary recommendations based on your individual health needs.

67. Apples baked with cinnamon

Ingredients:
- 4 medium-sized apples (choose a variety like Granny Smith or Honeycrisp)
- 1-2 tablespoons of lemon juice (optional, for preventing browning)
- 2 teaspoons of ground cinnamon
- 1-2 tablespoons of granulated sugar or sugar substitute (optional, adjust to taste)
- 1-2 tablespoons of unsalted butter or margarine (optional)

Instructions:

1. Preheat your oven to 375°F (190°C). Grease a baking dish with a small amount of butter or margarine, if using.

2. Wash the apples thoroughly under cold water and pat them dry with a paper towel.

3. Core the apples using an apple corer or a small knife, making sure to remove the seeds and stem.

4. If desired, you can peel the apples or leave the skins on for added fiber and texture.

5. Place the cored apples in the prepared baking dish. If using lemon juice, drizzle it over the apples to prevent browning.

6. In a small bowl, mix together the ground cinnamon and granulated sugar or sugar substitute, if using.

7. Sprinkle the cinnamon-sugar mixture evenly over the apples, making sure to coat them well.

8. If using, cut the unsalted butter or margarine into small pieces and dot the tops of the apples with it.

9. Cover the baking dish with aluminum foil and bake the apples in the preheated oven for about 25-30 minutes, or until they are tender.

10. Remove the foil and bake the apples for an additional 5-10 minutes, or until they are lightly golden brown and caramelized. Once baked, remove the apples from the oven and let them cool slightly before serving.

Enjoy these delicious baked apples with cinnamon as a kidney-friendly dessert or snack. They're naturally sweet and fragrant, with warm spices that complement the flavor of the apples perfectly. As always, consult with a healthcare professional or a registered dietitian for personalized dietary recommendations based on your individual health needs.

68. Fruit kabobs with yogurt dip

Ingredients:
- Assorted fresh fruits (such as strawberries, pineapple chunks, grapes, melon cubes, and kiwi slices)
- Wooden skewers or bamboo skewers
- 1 cup of plain Greek yogurt
- 1-2 tablespoons of honey or maple syrup (optional, for sweetening the yogurt dip)
- 1 teaspoon of vanilla extract (optional, for flavoring the yogurt dip)
- Fresh mint leaves for garnish (optional)

Instructions:

1. Wash and prepare the assorted fresh fruits. If needed, cut them into bite-sized pieces or slices.

2. Thread the prepared fruits onto wooden skewers, alternating between different types of fruits to create colorful kabobs. Leave a little space at the ends of the skewers for easy handling.

3. In a small bowl, mix together the plain Greek yogurt, honey or maple syrup (if using), and vanilla extract (if using). Stir until well combined. Taste and adjust the sweetness if necessary.

4. Transfer the yogurt dip to a serving bowl and garnish with fresh mint leaves, if desired.

5. Arrange the fruit kabobs on a serving platter or tray alongside the yogurt dip.

6. Serve the fruit kabobs with yogurt dip immediately and enjoy!

This kidney-friendly snack is packed with vitamins, minerals, and antioxidants from the fresh fruits, while the Greek yogurt provides protein and calcium. It's a perfect option for a light and nutritious treat. As always, consult with a healthcare professional or a registered dietitian for personalized dietary recommendations based on your individual health needs.

69. Frozen yogurt (low-sodium, low-phosphorus)

Ingredients:
- 2 cups of plain Greek yogurt (low-sodium and low-phosphorus)
- 2 tablespoons of honey or maple syrup (optional, for sweetness)
- 1 teaspoon of vanilla extract (optional, for flavor)
- Fresh fruit or nuts for topping (choose low-potassium options like berries or almonds)

Instructions:

1. In a mixing bowl, combine the plain Greek yogurt, honey or maple syrup (if using), and vanilla extract (if using). Stir until well combined. Taste and adjust sweetness if necessary.

2. If desired, you can blend the mixture in a blender or food processor for a smoother texture.

3. Pour the yogurt mixture into an ice cream maker and churn according to the manufacturer's instructions until it reaches a soft-serve consistency.

4. Transfer the frozen yogurt to a container with a lid and freeze for an additional 1-2 hours, or until it firms up.

5. Once the frozen yogurt is firm, scoop it into serving bowls or cones.

6. Top with fresh fruit or nuts for added flavor and texture.

7. Serve immediately and enjoy!

This kidney-friendly frozen yogurt is a delicious and nutritious treat, perfect for satisfying your sweet cravings while adhering to dietary restrictions. As always, consult with a healthcare professional or a registered dietitian for personalized dietary recommendations based on your individual health needs.

70. Peach sorbet

Ingredients:
- 4 ripe peaches, peeled, pitted, and chopped
- 1/2 cup of water
- 1/4 cup of granulated sugar or sugar substitute (adjust to taste)
- 1 tablespoon of lemon juice (optional, for added tartness)
- Fresh mint leaves for garnish (optional)

Instructions:
1. Place the chopped peaches, water, and granulated sugar or sugar substitute in a blender or food processor.

2. If using, add the lemon juice to the blender for added tartness.

3. Blend the ingredients until smooth and well combined. If the mixture is too thick, you can add a little more water to reach your desired consistency.

4. Taste the mixture and adjust the sweetness if necessary by adding more sugar or sugar substitute.

5. Once the sorbet mixture is smooth and sweetened to your liking, transfer it to a shallow dish or baking pan.

6. Place the dish or pan in the freezer and let the sorbet freeze for about 2-3 hours, or until it is firm.

7. Every 30 minutes during the freezing process, remove the sorbet from the freezer and stir it with a fork to break up any ice crystals and maintain a smooth texture.

8. Once the sorbet is frozen and has reached your desired consistency, remove it from the freezer.

9. Use a spoon or ice cream scoop to scoop the peach sorbet into serving bowls.

10. Garnish with fresh mint leaves if desired, and serve immediately.

Enjoy this homemade peach sorbet as a kidney-friendly dessert or treat. It's naturally sweet and packed with the flavors of ripe peaches. As always, consult with a healthcare professional or a registered dietitian for personalized dietary recommendations based on your individual health needs.

71. Chicken and broccoli casserole

Ingredients:
- 2 cups of cooked chicken breast, diced
- 2 cups of broccoli florets, steamed
- 1 cup of low-sodium chicken broth
- 1 cup of low-fat sour cream
- 1/2 cup of grated Parmesan cheese
- 1/4 cup of chopped onion
- 2 cloves of garlic, minced
- 2 tablespoons of olive oil
- 1 tablespoon of all-purpose flour
- 1/2 teaspoon of dried thyme
- Salt and pepper to taste
- Cooking spray

Instructions:

1. Preheat your oven to 375°F (190°C). Grease a casserole dish with cooking spray.

2. In a skillet, heat the olive oil over medium heat. Add the chopped onion and minced garlic, and sauté until softened, about 2-3 minutes.

3. Sprinkle the flour over the onion and garlic, and cook for another minute, stirring constantly.

4. Gradually add the chicken broth to the skillet, stirring constantly to prevent lumps from forming.

5. Bring the mixture to a simmer, then reduce the heat to low. Cook until the sauce thickens, about 2-3 minutes.

6. Stir in the low-fat sour cream, grated Parmesan cheese, dried thyme, salt, and pepper. Cook for an additional 2-3 minutes, until the cheese is melted and the sauce is smooth.

7. In a large mixing bowl, combine the cooked chicken breast and steamed broccoli florets.

8. Pour the sauce over the chicken and broccoli mixture, and toss until everything is well coated.

9. Transfer the mixture to the prepared casserole dish, spreading it out evenly.

10. Bake in the preheated oven for 25-30 minutes, or until the casserole is hot and bubbly.

11. Remove from the oven and let it cool for a few minutes before serving.

Enjoy this kidney-friendly chicken and broccoli casserole as a wholesome and satisfying meal. It's packed with protein from the chicken breast and nutrients from the broccoli, making it a nutritious choice for individuals with kidney disease. As always, consult with a healthcare professional or a registered dietitian for personalized dietary recommendations based on your individual health needs.

72. Fish tacos with cabbage slaw

Ingredients:
For the fish:
- 1 lb white fish fillets
  (such as cod, tilapia, or mahi-mahi)
- 1 tablespoon olive oil
- 1 teaspoon ground cumin
- 1 teaspoon chili powder
- Salt and pepper to taste

For the cabbage slaw:
- 2 cups shredded cabbage (green or purple)
- 1/4 cup chopped cilantro
- 1/4 cup plain Greek yogurt
- 1 tablespoon lime juice
- 1 tablespoon honey or maple syrup
(optional, for sweetness)
- Salt and pepper to taste

For serving:
- Corn tortillas
- Sliced avocado
- Lime wedges
- Hot sauce (optional)

Instructions:
1. Preheat your oven to 375°F (190°C).

2. In a small bowl, mix together the olive oil, ground cumin, chili powder, salt, and pepper.

3. Place the fish fillets on a baking sheet lined with parchment paper or aluminum foil.

4. Brush the spice mixture evenly over the fish fillets.

5. Bake in the preheated oven for 12-15 minutes, or until the fish is cooked through and flakes easily with a fork.

6. While the fish is baking, prepare the cabbage slaw. In a mixing bowl, combine the shredded cabbage, chopped cilantro, plain Greek yogurt, lime juice, honey or maple syrup (if using), salt, and pepper. Toss until well combined.

7. Warm the corn tortillas in a dry skillet or in the oven.

8. To assemble the tacos, place a spoonful of the cabbage slaw on each tortilla, followed by a piece of baked fish.

9. Top with sliced avocado and a squeeze of lime juice.

10. Serve the fish tacos with additional lime wedges and hot sauce on the side, if desired.

Enjoy these kidney-friendly fish tacos with cabbage slaw as a nutritious and delicious meal. The combination of flavorful spices, tender fish, crunchy cabbage slaw, and creamy avocado is sure to satisfy your taste buds. As always, consult with a healthcare professional or a registered dietitian for personalized dietary recommendations based on your individual health needs.

73. Barley and vegetable soup

Ingredients:
- 1 cup pearl barley
- 8 cups low-sodium vegetable broth
- 2 carrots, diced
- 2 celery stalks, diced
- 1 onion, diced
- 2 cloves garlic, minced
- 1 cup diced tomatoes (canned or fresh)
- 1 cup chopped spinach or kale
- 1 teaspoon dried thyme
- 1 teaspoon dried rosemary
- Salt and pepper to taste
- 2 tablespoons olive oil
- Fresh parsley for garnish (optional)

Instructions:
1. Rinse the pearl barley under cold water.

2. In a large pot, heat the olive oil over medium heat. Add the diced onion, carrots, and celery. Cook until the vegetables are softened, about 5-7 minutes.

3. Add the minced garlic, dried thyme, and dried rosemary to the pot. Cook for another 1-2 minutes until fragrant.

4. Pour in the vegetable broth and diced tomatoes. Bring the mixture to a boil.

5. Add the rinsed pearl barley to the pot. Reduce the heat to low, cover, and simmer for about 30-40 minutes, or until the barley is tender.

6. Stir in the chopped spinach or kale and cook for an additional 5 minutes until wilted.

7. Season the soup with salt and pepper to taste.

8. Ladle the soup into bowls and garnish with fresh parsley, if desired. Serve hot and enjoy!

This kidney-friendly barley and vegetable soup is packed with fiber, vitamins, and minerals. It's a comforting and nutritious meal option for individuals with kidney disease. As always, consult with a healthcare professional or a registered dietitian for personalized dietary recommendations based on your individual health needs.

74. Grilled turkey burgers with lettuce wraps

Ingredients:

For the turkey burgers:
- 1 lb ground turkey
- 1/4 cup finely chopped onion
- 2 cloves garlic, minced
- 1/4 cup chopped fresh parsley
- 1 teaspoon dried oregano
- 1 teaspoon dried basil
- 1/2 teaspoon salt
- 1/4 teaspoon black pepper
- Olive oil or cooking spray, for grilling

For serving:
- Large lettuce leaves (such as iceberg or butter lettuce)
- Sliced tomato
- Sliced red onion
- Sliced avocado
- Mustard or low-sodium ketchup (optional)

Instructions:

1. Preheat your grill to medium-high heat.

2. In a mixing bowl, combine the ground turkey, chopped onion, minced garlic, chopped parsley, dried oregano, dried basil, salt, and black pepper. Mix until well combined.

3. Divide the turkey mixture into 4 equal portions and shape each portion into a burger patty.

4. Lightly brush the grill grates with olive oil or spray with cooking spray to prevent sticking.

5. Place the turkey burger patties on the grill and cook for about 5-6 minutes on each side, or until cooked through and no longer pink in the center.

6. While the turkey burgers are cooking, prepare the lettuce wraps and toppings. Wash and dry the lettuce leaves, and slice the tomato, red onion, and avocado.

7. Once the turkey burgers are cooked, remove them from the grill and let them rest for a few minutes.

8. To assemble the lettuce wraps, place a turkey burger patty on each lettuce leaf and top with sliced tomato, red onion, and avocado. Add mustard or low-sodium ketchup if desired.

9. Fold the lettuce leaves around the burger patties to create wraps. Serve the grilled turkey burgers with lettuce wraps immediately and enjoy!

These kidney-friendly grilled turkey burgers with lettuce wraps are packed with protein and nutrients, making them a wholesome and satisfying meal option. Feel free to customize the toppings to suit your taste preferences. As always, consult with a healthcare professional or a registered dietitian for personalized dietary recommendations based on your individual health needs.

75. Ratatouille with fresh herbs

Ingredients:
- 1 eggplant, diced
- 2 zucchinis, diced
- 1 bell pepper (red, yellow, or green), diced
- 1 onion, diced
- 2 cloves garlic, minced
- 2 cups diced tomatoes (canned or fresh)
- 2 tablespoons tomato paste
- 1 teaspoon dried thyme
- 1 teaspoon dried oregano
- 1 teaspoon dried basil
- Salt and pepper to taste
- Olive oil for cooking
- Fresh herbs for garnish (such as chopped parsley, basil, or thyme)

Instructions:

1. Heat a couple of tablespoons of olive oil in a large skillet or pot over medium heat.

2. Add the diced onion to the skillet and cook until softened, about 5 minutes.

3. Add the minced garlic to the skillet and cook for an additional minute until fragrant.

4. Add the diced eggplant, zucchini, and bell pepper to the skillet. Cook, stirring occasionally, until the vegetables are slightly softened, about 5-7 minutes.

5. Stir in the diced tomatoes, tomato paste, dried thyme, dried oregano, and dried basil. Season with salt and pepper to taste.

6. Reduce the heat to low, cover the skillet, and let the ratatouille simmer for about 20-25 minutes, stirring occasionally, until the vegetables are tender and the flavors are well combined.

7. Once the ratatouille is cooked, remove it from the heat and let it cool slightly. Taste and adjust seasoning if necessary.

8. Serve the ratatouille garnished with fresh herbs, such as chopped parsley, basil, or thyme. Enjoy this kidney-friendly ratatouille as a flavorful side dish or main course.

This ratatouille with fresh herbs is packed with vitamins, minerals, and antioxidants from the variety of vegetables and herbs used. It's a delicious and nutritious option for individuals with kidney disease. As always, consult with a healthcare professional or a registered dietitian for personalized dietary recommendations based on your individual health needs.

76. Low-sodium black bean soup

Ingredients:
- 1 teaspoon ground cumin
- 1 teaspoon chili powder
- 1/2 teaspoon paprika
- Salt and pepper to taste
- 2 tablespoons olive oil
- Fresh cilantro for garnish (optional)
- Lime wedges for serving (optional)
- 2 cans (15 ounces each) of low-sodium black beans, drained and rinsed
- 1 onion, chopped
- 2 cloves garlic, minced
- 1 carrot, diced
- 1 stalk celery, diced
- 1 bell pepper (any color), diced
- 4 cups low-sodium vegetable broth

Instructions:

1. Heat the olive oil in a large pot over medium heat.

2. Add the chopped onion, minced garlic, diced carrot, diced celery, and diced bell pepper to the pot. Cook, stirring occasionally, until the vegetables are softened, about 5-7 minutes.

3. Stir in the ground cumin, chili powder, and paprika, and cook for an additional minute until fragrant.

4. Add the drained and rinsed black beans to the pot, along with the low-sodium vegetable broth.

5. Bring the soup to a simmer, then reduce the heat to low. Cover and let the soup simmer for about 15-20 minutes to allow the flavors to meld together.

6. Use an immersion blender or transfer a portion of the soup to a blender, and blend until smooth. Be careful when blending hot liquids.

7. Return the blended soup to the pot and stir to combine. If you prefer a chunkier texture, you can skip this step.

8. Season the soup with salt and pepper to taste, adjusting as needed. Serve the low-sodium black bean soup hot, garnished with fresh cilantro and lime wedges if desired.

This kidney-friendly black bean soup is rich in fiber, protein, and flavor, making it a nutritious and satisfying meal option. It's perfect for those looking to reduce their sodium intake without sacrificing taste. As always, consult with a healthcare professional or a registered dietitian for personalized dietary recommendations based on your individual health needs.

77. Turkey chili with bell peppers

Ingredients:
- 1 lb ground turkey
- 1 onion, diced
- 2 cloves garlic, minced
- 1 tablespoon chili powder
- 1 teaspoon ground cumin
- 1/2 teaspoon paprika
- Salt and pepper to taste
- Olive oil for cooking
- 2 bell peppers (any color), diced
- 1 can (15 ounces) low-sodium kidney beans, drained and rinsed
- 1 can (15 ounces) low-sodium diced tomatoes
- 1 cup low-sodium chicken or vegetable broth
- 2 tablespoons tomato paste
- Optional toppings: shredded cheese, chopped cilantro, diced avocado, Greek yogurt or sour cream

Instructions:

1. Heat a drizzle of olive oil in a large pot over medium heat.

2. Add the diced onion and minced garlic to the pot. Cook, stirring occasionally, until the onion is softened and translucent, about 5 minutes.

3. Add the ground turkey to the pot, breaking it apart with a spoon. Cook until the turkey is browned and cooked through, about 5-7 minutes.

4. Stir in the diced bell peppers and cook for another 3-4 minutes, until they begin to soften.

5. Add the low-sodium kidney beans, diced tomatoes, low-sodium chicken or vegetable broth, tomato paste, chili powder, ground cumin, paprika, salt, and pepper to the pot. Stir to combine.

6. Bring the chili to a simmer, then reduce the heat to low. Cover and let the chili simmer for about 20-25 minutes, stirring occasionally.

7. Taste and adjust the seasoning as needed, adding more salt and pepper if desired.

8. Serve the turkey chili hot, garnished with your choice of toppings such as shredded cheese, chopped cilantro, diced avocado, or Greek yogurt/sour cream.

This kidney-friendly turkey chili with bell peppers is hearty, flavorful, and packed with protein and nutrients. It's a comforting meal option that's perfect for chilly days. As always, consult with a healthcare professional or a registered dietitian for personalized dietary recommendations based on your individual health needs.

78. Grilled zucchini and squash

Ingredients:
- 2 medium zucchinis
- 2 medium yellow squash
- 2 tablespoons olive oil
- 2 cloves garlic, minced
- Salt and pepper to taste
- Fresh herbs for garnish (such as chopped parsley or basil)

Instructions:

1. Preheat your grill to medium-high heat.

2. Wash the zucchinis and yellow squash and pat them dry with a paper towel.

3. Slice the zucchinis and yellow squash into rounds, about 1/4 to 1/2 inch thick.

4. In a small bowl, mix together the olive oil and minced garlic.

5. Brush both sides of the zucchini and squash slices with the olive oil mixture.

6. Season the slices with salt and pepper to taste.

7. Place the zucchini and squash slices directly on the grill grates.

8. Grill for about 3-4 minutes on each side, or until they are tender and have grill marks.

9. Once grilled, remove the zucchini and squash slices from the grill and transfer them to a serving platter.

10. Garnish with fresh herbs, such as chopped parsley or basil, if desired.

11. Serve the grilled zucchini and squash hot as a side dish or accompaniment to your favorite grilled meats or seafood.

Enjoy this kidney-friendly grilled zucchini and squash as a flavorful and nutritious addition to your summer meals. They're packed with vitamins, minerals, and antioxidants, making them a healthy choice for individuals with kidney disease. As always, consult with a healthcare professional or a registered dietitian for personalized dietary recommendations based on your individual health needs.

79. Cauliflower rice stir-fry

Ingredients:
- 1 head of cauliflower
- 2 tablespoons olive oil or sesame oil
- 1 onion, diced
- 2 cloves garlic, minced
- 1 carrot, diced
- 1 bell pepper (any color), diced
- 1 cup chopped broccoli florets
- 1 cup chopped cabbage
- 2 tablespoons low-sodium soy sauce or tamari
- 1 tablespoon rice vinegar
- 1 teaspoon sesame seeds (optional)
- Salt and pepper to taste
- Green onions, chopped, for garnish (optional)

Instructions:
1. Remove the leaves and core from the cauliflower and cut it into florets. Place the cauliflower florets in a food processor and pulse until they resemble rice-like grains. Alternatively, you can grate the cauliflower using a box grater.

2. Heat the olive oil or sesame oil in a large skillet or wok over medium heat.

3. Add the diced onion and minced garlic to the skillet. Cook, stirring occasionally, until the onion is softened and translucent, about 5 minutes.

4. Add the diced carrot, bell pepper, chopped broccoli florets, and chopped cabbage to the skillet. Cook, stirring frequently, until the vegetables are tender-crisp, about 5-7 minutes.

5. Push the vegetables to one side of the skillet and add the riced cauliflower to the empty side. Cook the cauliflower, stirring occasionally, until it is tender, about 5 minutes.

6. Combine the cooked vegetables and cauliflower rice in the skillet. Stir in the low-sodium soy sauce or tamari and rice vinegar. Cook for an additional 2-3 minutes to allow the flavors to meld together.

7. Taste the stir-fry and adjust the seasoning with salt and pepper if necessary. Remove the skillet from the heat and transfer the cauliflower rice stir-fry to a serving dish. Garnish with sesame seeds and chopped green onions, if desired. Serve hot and enjoy!

This kidney-friendly cauliflower rice stir-fry is packed with vegetables and flavor, making it a nutritious and satisfying meal option. It's low in carbohydrates and suitable for individuals following a low-carb or keto diet as well. As always, consult with a healthcare professional or a registered dietitian for personalized dietary recommendations based on your individual health needs.

80. Broiled white fish with lemon and herbs

Ingredients:
- 4 white fish fillets (such as tilapia, cod, or sole)
- 2 tablespoons olive oil
- 2 cloves garlic, minced
- 2 tablespoons fresh lemon juice
- Zest of 1 lemon
- 2 tablespoons chopped fresh herbs (such as parsley, dill, or thyme)
- Salt and pepper to taste
- Lemon slices for garnish
- Fresh herbs for garnish

Instructions:

1. Preheat your broiler on high heat and position the oven rack about 6 inches below the broiler element.

2. Pat the fish fillets dry with paper towels and place them on a baking sheet lined with aluminum foil or parchment paper.

3. In a small bowl, whisk together the olive oil, minced garlic, fresh lemon juice, lemon zest, chopped fresh herbs, salt, and pepper.

4. Drizzle the lemon and herb mixture evenly over the fish fillets, using a brush or spoon to coat them well.

5. Place the baking sheet with the fish fillets under the preheated broiler.

6. Broil the fish for 6-8 minutes, or until it is opaque and flakes easily with a fork. The cooking time may vary depending on the thickness of the fish fillets, so keep an eye on them to prevent overcooking.

7. Once the fish is cooked through, remove it from the oven and transfer it to serving plates.

8. Garnish the broiled fish with lemon slices and fresh herbs. Serve hot and enjoy!

This broiled white fish with lemon and herbs is light, flavorful, and incredibly easy to make. It's perfect for a quick weeknight dinner or a special occasion meal. Pair it with your favorite side dishes, such as steamed vegetables or a leafy green salad, for a complete and balanced meal. As always, consult with a healthcare professional or a registered dietitian for personalized dietary recommendations based on your individual health needs.

81. Chicken fajitas with bell peppers and onions

Ingredients:
For the chicken marinade:
- 1 lb boneless,
skinless chicken breasts, thinly sliced
- 2 tablespoons olive oil
- 2 cloves garlic, minced
- 1 teaspoon chili powder
- 1 teaspoon ground cumin
- 1/2 teaspoon paprika
- 1/2 teaspoon dried oregano
- Juice of 1 lime
- Salt and pepper to taste

For the fajitas:
- 2 bell peppers (any color), thinly sliced
- 1 onion, thinly sliced
- 2 tablespoons olive oil
- Salt and pepper to taste
- 8 small flour tortillas
- Optional toppings: shredded cheese, sour cream, guacamole, salsa, chopped cilantro, lime wedges

Instructions:
1. In a mixing bowl, combine the olive oil, minced garlic, chili powder, ground cumin, paprika, dried oregano, lime juice, salt, and pepper. Mix well.

2. Add the sliced chicken breasts to the marinade and toss to coat. Cover and refrigerate for at least 30 minutes, or up to 4 hours, to allow the flavors to meld. Heat 1 tablespoon of olive oil in a large skillet over medium-high heat.

3. Add the sliced bell peppers and onions to the skillet. Cook, stirring occasionally, until the vegetables are tender and slightly charred, about 5-7 minutes. Season with salt and pepper to taste. Remove the cooked vegetables from the skillet and set aside. In the same skillet, heat the remaining tablespoon of olive oil over medium-high heat.

4. Add the marinated chicken slices to the skillet, spreading them out in an even layer. Cook for 5-7 minutes, stirring occasionally, until the chicken is cooked through and browned on the outside.

5. Once the chicken is cooked, return the cooked bell peppers and onions to the skillet. Stir to combine and heat through. Warm the flour tortillas in a dry skillet or in the microwave according to the package instructions.

6. Serve the chicken fajitas hot, spooning the chicken and vegetable mixture onto the warm tortillas.

7. Garnish with your choice of toppings, such as shredded cheese, sour cream, guacamole, salsa, chopped cilantro, and lime wedges. Roll up the tortillas and enjoy your delicious chicken fajitas!

82. Mushroom and spinach frittata

Ingredients:
- 8 large eggs
- 1/4 cup milk or heavy cream
- Salt and pepper to taste
- 1 tablespoon olive oil
- 8 ounces mushrooms, sliced
- 2 cups fresh spinach, chopped
- 1 small onion, diced
- 2 cloves garlic, minced
- 1/2 cup shredded cheese (such as cheddar, mozzarella, or Swiss)
- Fresh herbs for garnish (such as chopped parsley or chives)

Instructions:

1. Preheat your oven to 350°F (175°C).

2. In a mixing bowl, whisk together the eggs, milk or heavy cream, salt, and pepper until well combined. Set aside.

3. Heat the olive oil in a large oven-safe skillet over medium heat.

4. Add the diced onion to the skillet and cook until softened and translucent, about 5 minutes.

5. Add the sliced mushrooms to the skillet and cook until they are tender and golden brown, about 5-7 minutes.

6. Stir in the minced garlic and chopped spinach, and cook for another 2-3 minutes until the spinach is wilted. Spread the cooked vegetables evenly across the skillet.

7. Pour the egg mixture over the vegetables in the skillet, ensuring that the eggs cover the vegetables evenly. Sprinkle the shredded cheese over the top of the frittata.

8. Transfer the skillet to the preheated oven and bake for 20-25 minutes, or until the eggs are set and the top of the frittata is lightly golden brown.

9. Once the frittata is cooked through, remove it from the oven and let it cool slightly.. Garnish the frittata with fresh herbs, such as chopped parsley or chives. Slice the frittata into wedges and serve warm.

This mushroom and spinach frittata is a versatile dish that can be enjoyed for breakfast, brunch, lunch, or dinner. It's packed with protein from the eggs and nutrients from the vegetables, making it a nutritious and satisfying meal option. As always, consult with a healthcare professional or a registered dietitian for personalized dietary recommendations based on your individual health needs.

83. Baked sweet potato with cinnamon

Ingredients:
- 2 medium sweet potatoes
- 1 tablespoon olive oil or melted butter (optional)
- Ground cinnamon, to taste
- Salt, to taste

Instructions:
1. Preheat your oven to 400°F (200°C).

2. Wash the sweet potatoes and scrub them clean. Pat dry with a paper towel.

3. Pierce each sweet potato several times with a fork to create small holes.

4. Rub the sweet potatoes with olive oil or melted butter, if using.

5. Sprinkle ground cinnamon evenly over the sweet potatoes, adjusting the amount to your taste preferences.

6. Season the sweet potatoes with a pinch of salt.

7. Place the sweet potatoes on a baking sheet lined with parchment paper or aluminum foil.

8. Bake in the preheated oven for 45-60 minutes, or until the sweet potatoes are tender and can be easily pierced with a fork.

9. Once baked, remove the sweet potatoes from the oven and let them cool slightly.

10. Serve the baked sweet potatoes with cinnamon hot, optionally topped with additional butter or a sprinkle of brown sugar for extra sweetness.

Enjoy these delicious and nutritious baked sweet potatoes with cinnamon as a side dish or light meal. They're packed with vitamins, minerals, and fiber, making them a healthy choice for any occasion. As always, feel free to adjust the seasoning and toppings according to your preferences.

84. Vegetable paella with saffron

Ingredients:
- 1 cup paella rice (such as Arborio or Valencia)
- 2 cups vegetable broth
- 1 onion, chopped
- 2 cloves garlic, minced
- 1 red bell pepper, diced
- 1 yellow bell pepper, diced
- 1 zucchini, diced
- 1 cup cherry tomatoes, halved
- 1/2 cup green peas (fresh or frozen)
- 1/2 teaspoon saffron threads
- 1 teaspoon smoked paprika
- Salt and pepper to taste
- 2 tablespoons olive oil
- Lemon wedges for serving
- Fresh parsley for garnish (optional)

Instructions:
1. In a small bowl, crush the saffron threads and soak them in 1/4 cup warm water for about 10 minutes.

2. In a large skillet or paella pan, heat the olive oil over medium heat.

3. Add the chopped onion and minced garlic to the skillet. Cook until the onion is softened and translucent, about 5 minutes.

4. Stir in the diced bell peppers and diced zucchini. Cook for another 5 minutes, until the vegetables are slightly softened.

5. Add the paella rice to the skillet and stir to coat the rice with the oil and vegetables.

6. Pour the vegetable broth and saffron-infused water into the skillet. Add the smoked paprika, salt, and pepper. Stir to combine.

7. Bring the mixture to a simmer, then reduce the heat to low. Cover and cook for about 15-20 minutes, or until the rice is cooked through and most of the liquid is absorbed.

8. Stir in the halved cherry tomatoes and green peas. Cook for an additional 5 minutes, until the tomatoes are softened and the peas are heated through.

9. Taste and adjust the seasoning if necessary. Remove the skillet from the heat and let it rest for a few minutes before serving. Garnish the vegetable paella with fresh parsley, if desired, and serve with lemon wedges on the side.

Enjoy this flavorful and colorful vegetable paella with saffron as a satisfying vegetarian meal. It's perfect for sharing with family and friends and can be customized with your favorite vegetables and herbs. As always, feel free to adjust the ingredients and seasonings according to your preferences.

85. Shrimp scampi with zucchini noodles

Ingredients:
- 1 lb shrimp, peeled and deveined
- 4 medium zucchini
- 4 cloves garlic, minced
- 2 tablespoons olive oil
- 2 tablespoons unsalted butter
- 1/4 cup dry white wine (optional)
- Juice of 1 lemon
- Salt and pepper to taste
- Crushed red pepper flakes (optional)
- Chopped fresh parsley for garnish
- Grated Parmesan cheese for serving (optional)

Instructions:
1. Using a spiralizer or vegetable peeler, create zucchini noodles (zoodles) from the zucchini. Set aside.

2. In a large skillet, heat the olive oil and butter over medium heat.

3. Add the minced garlic to the skillet and sauté for about 1 minute until fragrant.

4. Add the shrimp to the skillet and cook for 2-3 minutes per side until pink and cooked through. Remove the shrimp from the skillet and set aside.

5. If using, pour the white wine into the skillet and let it simmer for 1-2 minutes to reduce slightly.

6. Add the zucchini noodles to the skillet and toss to coat in the garlic butter mixture. Cook for 2-3 minutes until the zucchini noodles are tender but still slightly crisp.

7. Return the cooked shrimp to the skillet with the zucchini noodles.

8. Squeeze the lemon juice over the shrimp and zucchini noodles. Season with salt, pepper, and crushed red pepper flakes to taste.

9. Toss everything together until well combined and heated through. Garnish the shrimp scampi with chopped fresh parsley. Serve hot, optionally topped with grated Parmesan cheese.

Enjoy this light and flavorful shrimp scampi with zucchini noodles as a healthy and satisfying meal option. It's quick and easy to make, perfect for busy weeknights!

86. Stuffed cabbage rolls with ground turkey

Ingredients:
- 1 head of cabbage
- 1 lb ground turkey
- 1 cup cooked rice (white or brown)
- 1 onion, finely chopped
- 2 cloves garlic, minced
- 1 can (14.5 oz) diced tomatoes
- 1 tablespoon tomato paste
- 1 teaspoon dried thyme
- 1 teaspoon dried oregano
- Salt and pepper to taste
- Olive oil for cooking
- 2 cups low-sodium chicken or vegetable broth
- Fresh parsley for garnish (optional)

Instructions:

1. Preheat your oven to 350°F (175°C).

2. Bring a large pot of water to a boil. Remove the core from the cabbage and carefully separate the leaves. Blanch the cabbage leaves in the boiling water for 2-3 minutes, until they are softened. Remove the leaves from the water and set aside to cool.

3. In a large skillet, heat a drizzle of olive oil over medium heat. Add the chopped onion and minced garlic to the skillet and cook until softened and translucent, about 5 minutes.

4. Add the ground turkey to the skillet and cook until browned, breaking it apart with a spoon as it cooks.

5. Stir in the cooked rice, diced tomatoes, tomato paste, dried thyme, dried oregano, salt, and pepper. Cook for another 2-3 minutes until heated through and well combined.

6. Place a cabbage leaf on a flat surface. Spoon a portion of the turkey mixture onto the center of the leaf. Roll up the leaf, tucking in the sides, to form a cabbage roll. Repeat with the remaining cabbage leaves and turkey mixture.

7. Place the stuffed cabbage rolls seam side down in a large baking dish. Pour the chicken or vegetable broth over the cabbage rolls.

8. Cover the baking dish with aluminum foil and bake in the preheated oven for 45-50 minutes, until the cabbage rolls are cooked through and tender.

9. Remove the foil from the baking dish and garnish the stuffed cabbage rolls with fresh parsley, if desired. Serve hot and enjoy!

These stuffed cabbage rolls with ground turkey are a comforting and nutritious meal option. They're packed with protein, fiber, and flavor, making them a satisfying dish for any occasion. As always, feel free to customize the recipe with your favorite herbs and spices.

87. Chicken salad with grapes and walnuts

Ingredients:
- 2 cups cooked chicken breast, shredded or diced
- 1 cup red seedless grapes, halved
- 1/2 cup walnuts, chopped
- 1/4 cup celery, diced
- 1/4 cup red onion, finely chopped
- 1/4 cup mayonnaise
- 1 tablespoon lemon juice
- 1 tablespoon Dijon mustard
- Salt and pepper to taste
- Lettuce leaves, for serving (optional)

Instructions:

1. In a large mixing bowl, combine the cooked chicken breast, halved grapes, chopped walnuts, diced celery, and finely chopped red onion.

2. In a small bowl, whisk together the mayonnaise, lemon juice, and Dijon mustard until well combined.

3. Pour the dressing over the chicken salad mixture and toss until everything is evenly coated.

4. Season the chicken salad with salt and pepper to taste.

5. Cover the bowl and refrigerate the chicken salad for at least 30 minutes to allow the flavors to meld together.

6. When ready to serve, line a serving platter or individual plates with lettuce leaves, if using.

7. Scoop the chilled chicken salad onto the lettuce leaves and garnish with additional chopped walnuts and grapes, if desired.

8. Serve the chicken salad immediately and enjoy!

This chicken salad with grapes and walnuts is a delicious and refreshing dish, perfect for lunch, dinner, or as a light meal any time of the day. It's packed with protein, healthy fats, and a burst of sweetness from the grapes, making it a satisfying and nutritious option. Feel free to customize the recipe by adding your favorite herbs or spices.

88. Pumpkin soup with nutmeg

Ingredients:
- 2 tablespoons olive oil
- 1 onion, diced
- 2 cloves garlic, minced
- 1 teaspoon ground nutmeg
- 1/2 teaspoon ground cinnamon
- 1/4 teaspoon ground ginger
- 1/4 teaspoon ground cloves
- 4 cups pumpkin puree (canned or homemade)
- 4 cups vegetable broth
- Salt and pepper to taste
- 1/2 cup heavy cream (optional)
- Roasted pumpkin seeds for garnish (optional)
- Fresh parsley or chives for garnish (optional)

Instructions:

1. Heat the olive oil in a large pot over medium heat.

2. Add the diced onion to the pot and cook until softened and translucent, about 5 minutes.

3. Stir in the minced garlic, ground nutmeg, ground cinnamon, ground ginger, and ground cloves. Cook for another minute until fragrant.

4. Add the pumpkin puree and vegetable broth to the pot. Stir to combine.

5. Bring the soup to a simmer, then reduce the heat to low. Cover and let the soup simmer for about 15-20 minutes to allow the flavors to meld together.

6. Use an immersion blender or transfer the soup to a blender, and blend until smooth. Be careful when blending hot liquids.

7. Once the soup is blended, return it to the pot if necessary. Season with salt and pepper to taste.

8. If using heavy cream, stir it into the soup until well combined. Heat the soup for a few more minutes until warmed through.

9. Ladle the pumpkin soup into bowls and garnish with roasted pumpkin seeds, fresh parsley, or chives if desired. Serve hot and enjoy!

This pumpkin soup with nutmeg is creamy, comforting, and full of warm fall flavors. It's perfect for a cozy night in or as a starter for your holiday meal. Feel free to adjust the seasoning and consistency according to your taste preferences.

89. Chicken and wild rice casserole

Ingredients:
- 1 cup wild rice blend
- 2 cups water or chicken broth
- 2 tablespoons olive oil
- 1 onion, diced
- 2 cloves garlic, minced
- 2 carrots, diced
- 2 celery stalks, diced
- 2 cups cooked chicken breast, shredded or diced
- 1/2 cup frozen peas
- 1/2 cup frozen corn
- 1 teaspoon dried thyme
- 1 teaspoon dried parsley
- Salt and pepper to taste
- 1/2 cup shredded cheese (such as cheddar or mozzarella)
- 1/4 cup grated Parmesan cheese
- 1/4 cup breadcrumbs (optional)
- Fresh parsley for garnish (optional)

Instructions:

1. Preheat your oven to 350°F (175°C).

2. In a saucepan, combine the wild rice blend and water or chicken broth. Bring to a boil, then reduce the heat to low, cover, and simmer for 45-50 minutes, or until the rice is tender and all the liquid is absorbed. Remove from heat and set aside.

3. In a large skillet, heat the olive oil over medium heat. Add the diced onion and cook until softened and translucent, about 5 minutes.

4. Add the minced garlic, diced carrots, and diced celery to the skillet. Cook for another 5 minutes, until the vegetables are tender.

5. Stir in the cooked chicken breast, frozen peas, frozen corn, dried thyme, dried parsley, salt, and pepper. Cook for 2-3 minutes until heated through and well combined.

6. In a large mixing bowl, combine the cooked wild rice and chicken-vegetable mixture. Stir until evenly mixed.

7. Transfer the mixture to a greased baking dish and spread it out evenly. Sprinkle shredded cheese and grated Parmesan cheese over the top of the casserole.

8. If using breadcrumbs, sprinkle them evenly over the cheese layer.

9. Cover the baking dish with aluminum foil and bake in the preheated oven for 20-25 minutes.

10. Remove the foil and bake for an additional 5-10 minutes, until the cheese is melted and bubbly. Garnish with fresh parsley, if desired, before serving.

90. Steamed mussels with garlic and parsley

Ingredients:
- 2 lbs fresh mussels, cleaned and debearded
- 2 tablespoons olive oil
- 4 cloves garlic, minced
- 1/2 cup dry white wine
- 1/4 cup chopped fresh parsley
- Salt and pepper to taste
- Lemon wedges for serving
- Crusty bread for serving

Instructions:
1. Clean the mussels under cold running water, scrubbing off any dirt or debris. Remove the beards (the thread-like appendages) by pulling them gently towards the hinge of the shell. Discard any mussels with cracked shells or that do not close when tapped.

2. In a large pot or Dutch oven, heat the olive oil over medium heat. Add the minced garlic and sauté for 1-2 minutes until fragrant.

3. Pour the dry white wine into the pot and bring it to a simmer.

4. Add the cleaned mussels to the pot and cover with a lid. Steam the mussels for 5-7 minutes, shaking the pot occasionally, until the mussels have opened.

5. Discard any mussels that have not opened after cooking.

6. Once the mussels are cooked, remove the pot from the heat.

7. Sprinkle chopped fresh parsley over the steamed mussels and season with salt and pepper to taste.

8. Serve the steamed mussels with garlic and parsley immediately, with lemon wedges on the side for squeezing over the mussels.

9. Enjoy the mussels with crusty bread for soaking up the delicious broth.

This steamed mussels with garlic and parsley recipe is simple yet elegant, perfect for a special dinner or entertaining guests. It's a classic dish that highlights the natural flavor of the mussels, enhanced by the garlic, parsley, and white wine broth. Enjoy!

91. Strawberry and banana smoothie (using water or almond milk)

Ingredients:
- 2 cups old-fashioned oats
- 1/2 cup chopped nuts (such as almonds, pecans, or walnuts)
- 1/2 cup dried fruit (such as raisins, cranberries, or chopped apricots)
- 1/4 cup honey
- 1/4 cup peanut butter (or other nut butter)
- 1 tsp vanilla extract
- 1/4 tsp salt

Instructions:
1. Preheat your oven to 325°F. Line an 8x8-inch baking pan with parchment paper, leaving some overhang on the sides for easy removal.

2. In a large bowl, combine the oats, chopped nuts, and dried fruit. Stir to mix well.

3. In a small saucepan, heat the honey and peanut butter over medium heat, stirring constantly, until the mixture is smooth and well combined, about 2-3 minutes.

4. Remove the honey-peanut butter mixture from the heat and stir in the vanilla extract and salt.

5. Pour the honey-peanut butter mixture over the oat mixture and stir until everything is evenly coated.

6. Transfer the granola bar mixture to the prepared baking pan and press it down firmly and evenly with a spatula or your hands.

7. Bake for 20-25 minutes, until the edges are lightly golden brown.

8. Allow the granola bars to cool completely in the pan, then use the parchment paper to lift them out. Cut into bars or squares.

9. Store the homemade granola bars in an airtight container at room temperature for up to 1 week.

These homemade granola bars are a great snack option for bachelor men because they're:

- Easy to make with simple, wholesome ingredients
- Customizable with different nuts, dried fruits, and nut butters
- Portable and perfect for on-the-go snacking
- Healthier and more cost-effective than store-bought granola bars

92. Green smoothie with kale, cucumber, and apple

Ingredients:
- 1 cup chopped kale leaves, stems removed
- 1/2 cucumber, peeled and chopped
- 1 apple, cored and chopped
- 1/2 cup water or coconut water
- 1/2 cup ice cubes (optional)
- Juice of 1/2 lemon (optional, for added tanginess)
- Honey or maple syrup to taste (optional, for added sweetness)

Instructions:

1. Place the chopped kale leaves, cucumber, apple, water or coconut water, and ice cubes (if using) in a blender.

2. Squeeze in the juice of half a lemon for added tanginess, if desired.

3. If you prefer a sweeter smoothie, add honey or maple syrup to taste.

4. Blend the ingredients on high speed until smooth and creamy, scraping down the sides of the blender as needed.

5. Once the green smoothie reaches your desired consistency, taste and adjust the sweetness or tartness if necessary.

6. Pour the green smoothie into glasses and serve immediately.

This green smoothie with kale, cucumber, and apple is packed with nutrients, including vitamins, minerals, and antioxidants. It's a refreshing and hydrating drink that's perfect for starting your day or as a midday pick-me-up. Enjoy!

93. Blueberry and spinach smoothie

Ingredients:
- 1 cup fresh or frozen blueberries
- 1 cup fresh spinach leaves
- 1 ripe banana, peeled and sliced
- 1/2 cup Greek yogurt (plain or vanilla)
- 1/2 cup almond milk or any milk of your choice
- 1 tablespoon honey or maple syrup (optional, for added sweetness)
- Ice cubes (optional, for a colder smoothie)

Instructions:

1. Place the blueberries, spinach leaves, sliced banana, Greek yogurt, almond milk, and honey or maple syrup (if using) in a blender.

2. If you prefer a colder smoothie, add a handful of ice cubes to the blender.

3. Blend the ingredients on high speed until smooth and creamy, scraping down the sides of the blender as needed.

4. Once the blueberry and spinach smoothie reaches your desired consistency, taste and adjust the sweetness if necessary.

5. Pour the smoothie into glasses and serve immediately.

This blueberry and spinach smoothie is not only delicious but also packed with vitamins, minerals, and antioxidants from the blueberries and spinach. It's a nutritious and refreshing drink that's perfect for breakfast, a snack, or anytime you need a boost of energy. Enjoy!

94. Herbal iced tea with lemon

Ingredients:
- 4 cups water
- 4 herbal tea bags (such as chamomile, peppermint, or herbal berry)
- 1 lemon, thinly sliced
- Ice cubes
- Fresh mint leaves for garnish (optional)
- Honey or sweetener of choice (optional)

Instructions:
1. Bring 4 cups of water to a boil in a pot or kettle.

2. Once the water reaches a boil, remove it from heat and add the herbal tea bags to the pot.

3. Let the tea steep for about 5-7 minutes, or according to the instructions on the tea bags.

4. Once the tea has steeped, remove the tea bags from the pot and discard them.

5. Transfer the brewed tea to a heatproof pitcher and let it cool to room temperature.

6. Once the tea has cooled, place it in the refrigerator to chill for at least 1 hour, or until cold.
7. When ready to serve, fill glasses with ice cubes and pour the chilled herbal tea over the ice.

8. Add a few slices of lemon to each glass of iced tea for added flavor.

9. If desired, sweeten the iced tea with honey or your preferred sweetener.

10. Garnish the glasses with fresh mint leaves for a pop of color and additional flavor.

11. Stir the iced tea gently to combine all the ingredients.

12. Serve immediately and enjoy the refreshing herbal iced tea with lemon on a hot day!

This herbal iced tea with lemon is a delightful and hydrating beverage that's perfect for staying cool and refreshed during the summer months. Feel free to experiment with different herbal tea flavors and adjust the sweetness to suit your taste preferences. Cheers!

95. Pineapple and mint infused water

Ingredients:
- 1/2 cup fresh pineapple chunks
- 4-6 fresh mint leaves
- 4 cups water
- Ice cubes (optional)

Instructions:

1. Place the fresh pineapple chunks and mint leaves in a pitcher.

2. Using a muddler or the back of a spoon, gently press down on the pineapple and mint to release their flavors.

3. Add the water to the pitcher, covering the pineapple and mint completely.

4. If desired, add ice cubes to the pitcher to chill the infused water further.

5. Stir the ingredients gently to combine.

6. Let the infused water sit in the refrigerator for at least 1 hour to allow the flavors to meld together.

7. Serve the pineapple and mint infused water in glasses over ice, if desired.

8. Garnish each glass with a sprig of fresh mint for an extra touch of freshness.

9. Enjoy this refreshing and hydrating pineapple and mint infused water anytime you need a flavorful and healthy beverage option!

This pineapple and mint infused water is a delicious and refreshing drink that's perfect for staying hydrated on hot days or as a flavorful alternative to plain water. Experiment with different fruit and herb combinations to create your own custom infused water recipes. Cheers to good hydration!

96. Low-sodium vegetable juice

Ingredients:
- 4 large tomatoes, roughly chopped
- 2 large carrots, peeled and chopped
- 2 celery stalks, chopped
- 1 red bell pepper, seeded and chopped
- 1 cucumber, peeled and chopped
- 1/2 small onion, chopped
- 2 cloves garlic, minced
- 1 tablespoon fresh lemon juice
- 1 tablespoon fresh parsley, chopped
- 1/4 teaspoon ground black pepper
- Dash of hot sauce (optional)
- Water, as needed

Instructions:
1. In a blender or food processor, combine the chopped tomatoes, carrots, celery, red bell pepper, cucumber, onion, and garlic.

2. Add the fresh lemon juice, chopped parsley, ground black pepper, and hot sauce (if using).

3. Blend the ingredients on high speed until smooth and well combined. If the mixture is too thick, add water gradually until you reach your desired consistency.

4. Once the vegetable juice reaches the desired consistency, taste and adjust the seasoning if necessary.

5. Pour the vegetable juice through a fine mesh strainer or cheesecloth to remove any pulp and solids, if desired.

6. Transfer the strained vegetable juice to a pitcher or glass bottles and refrigerate until chilled.

7. Serve the low-sodium vegetable juice cold over ice, if desired.

8. Enjoy this refreshing and nutritious beverage as a healthy snack or part of your daily routine!

This low-sodium vegetable juice is packed with vitamins, minerals, and antioxidants from a variety of colorful vegetables. It's a flavorful and hydrating option that's perfect for anyone looking to reduce their sodium intake without compromising on taste. Feel free to customize the recipe by adding your favorite herbs or spices. Cheers to good health!

97. Watermelon and mint smoothie

Ingredients:

- 2 cups cubed seedless watermelon
- 1/2 cup plain Greek yogurt
- 1 tablespoon honey or maple syrup (optional, for added sweetness)
- 4-6 fresh mint leaves
- 1/2 cup ice cubes

Instructions:

1. Place the cubed watermelon, Greek yogurt, honey or maple syrup (if using), and fresh mint leaves in a blender.

2. Add the ice cubes to the blender.

3. Blend the ingredients on high speed until smooth and creamy, scraping down the sides of the blender as needed.

4. Once the watermelon and mint smoothie reaches your desired consistency, taste and adjust the sweetness if necessary.

5. Pour the smoothie into glasses and serve immediately.

This watermelon and mint smoothie is a delicious and hydrating beverage that's perfect for hot summer days or anytime you need a refreshing pick-me-up. It's packed with vitamins, minerals, and antioxidants from the watermelon and fresh mint leaves, making it a healthy and satisfying option for breakfast, a snack, or dessert. Enjoy!

98. Berry and almond milk smoothie

Ingredients:

- 1 cup mixed berries (such as strawberries, blueberries, raspberries, or blackberries), fresh
or frozen
- 1 ripe banana, peeled and sliced
- 1 cup unsweetened almond milk (or any milk of your choice)
- 1 tablespoon almond butter or almond meal
- 1 tablespoon honey or maple syrup (optional, for added sweetness)
- Ice cubes (optional, for a colder smoothie)

Instructions:

1. Place the mixed berries, sliced banana, almond milk, almond butter or almond meal, and
honey or maple syrup (if using) in a blender.

2. If you prefer a colder smoothie, add a handful of ice cubes to the blender.

3. Blend the ingredients on high speed until smooth and creamy, scraping down the sides of
the blender as needed.

4. Once the berry and almond milk smoothie reaches your desired consistency, taste and
adjust the sweetness if necessary.

5. Pour the smoothie into glasses and serve immediately.

*This berry and almond milk smoothie is packed with antioxidants, vitamins, and minerals
from the mixed berries and almond milk. It's a nutritious and delicious beverage that's
perfect for breakfast, a snack, or post-workout fuel. Feel free to customize the recipe by
using your favorite berries or adding additional ingredients like spinach, protein powder,
or flaxseeds. Enjoy!*

99. Carrot and ginger juice

Ingredients:
- 4 large carrots, peeled and chopped
- 1-inch piece of fresh ginger, peeled and chopped
- 1/2 lemon, juiced
- 1-2 tablespoons honey or maple syrup (optional, for added sweetness)
- 2 cups water
- Ice cubes (optional, for a colder juice)

Instructions:

1. Place the chopped carrots and ginger in a blender or juicer.

2. Add the lemon juice and honey or maple syrup (if using) to the blender.

3. Pour in the water.

4. If using a blender, blend the ingredients on high speed until smooth. If using a juicer, process the carrots and ginger according to the manufacturer's instructions.

5. Once the carrot and ginger mixture is smooth, pour it through a fine mesh strainer or cheesecloth to remove any pulp.

6. Transfer the strained juice to a pitcher or glass bottles.

7. If desired, add ice cubes to the pitcher to chill the juice further.

8. Stir the juice gently to combine.

9. Serve the carrot and ginger juice cold over ice, if desired.

This carrot and ginger juice is a refreshing and invigorating beverage that's packed with vitamins, minerals, and antioxidants. It's perfect for boosting your immune system, aiding digestion, and providing a natural energy boost. Enjoy this nutritious juice any time of day for a refreshing pick-me-up!

100. Cucumber and lime infused water

Ingredients:
- 1 cucumber, thinly sliced
- 1 lime, thinly sliced
- 4 cups water
- Ice cubes

Instructions:

1. Place the sliced cucumber and lime in a pitcher.

2. Fill the pitcher with 4 cups of water.

3. Add ice cubes to the pitcher to chill the infused water further.

4. Stir the ingredients gently to combine.

5. Let the infused water sit in the refrigerator for at least 1 hour to allow the flavors to meld together.

6. Serve the cucumber and lime infused water cold over ice.

This cucumber and lime infused water is a refreshing and hydrating beverage that's perfect for staying cool and refreshed on hot days. It's naturally flavored and contains no added sugars or artificial ingredients, making it a healthy alternative to sugary drinks. Enjoy this delicious infused water any time you need a flavorful and thirst-quenching beverage!

101. Arugula salad with pears and walnuts

Ingredients:
- 4 cups fresh arugula leaves, washed and dried
- 2 ripe pears, thinly sliced
- 1/2 cup walnuts, chopped
- 1/4 cup crumbled feta cheese (optional)
- 2 tablespoons extra virgin olive oil
- 1 tablespoon balsamic vinegar
- 1 teaspoon honey or maple syrup (optional, for added sweetness)
- Salt and pepper to taste

Instructions:

1. In a large salad bowl, add the fresh arugula leaves.

2. Arrange the thinly sliced pears on top of the arugula.

3. Sprinkle the chopped walnuts (and crumbled feta cheese, if using) over the salad.

4. In a small bowl, whisk together the extra virgin olive oil, balsamic vinegar, honey or maple syrup (if using), salt, and pepper to make the dressing.

5. Drizzle the dressing over the salad just before serving.

6. Toss the salad gently to coat the ingredients evenly with the dressing.

7. Serve the arugula salad with pears and walnuts immediately as a refreshing and nutritious appetizer or side dish.

This arugula salad with pears and walnuts is a delicious combination of flavors and textures. The peppery arugula, sweet pears, crunchy walnuts, and tangy dressing create a delightful harmony of tastes that's sure to please your palate. Enjoy this salad as a light and satisfying meal any time of the year!

102. Beet and goat cheese salad

Ingredients:
- 4 medium-sized beets, cooked, peeled, and sliced
- 4 cups mixed salad greens (such as arugula, spinach, or mixed greens)
- 1/2 cup crumbled goat cheese
- 1/4 cup chopped walnuts or pecans (optional, for added crunch)
- Balsamic glaze or vinaigrette dressing

Instructions:
1. If you haven't already, cook the beets until tender, either by boiling, roasting, or steaming them. Once cooked, allow them to cool slightly before peeling and slicing them into thin rounds.

2. Arrange the mixed salad greens on a large serving platter or individual plates.

3. Place the sliced beets on top of the salad greens.

4. Sprinkle the crumbled goat cheese evenly over the salad.

5. If using, scatter the chopped walnuts or pecans on top of the salad for added crunch.

6. Drizzle balsamic glaze or vinaigrette dressing over the salad just before serving. Alternatively, you can serve the dressing on the side and let guests dress their own salads according to their preference.

7. Serve the beet and goat cheese salad immediately as a delightful and colorful appetizer or side dish.

This beet and goat cheese salad is a wonderful combination of earthy beets, creamy goat cheese, and crisp greens. The addition of nuts provides extra texture and flavor, while the balsamic glaze or vinaigrette dressing ties everything together beautifully. Enjoy this salad as a light and refreshing starter or side dish for any meal!

103. Farro salad with cranberries and pecans

Ingredients:
- 1 cup farro, rinsed
- 2 cups water or vegetable broth
- 1/2 cup dried cranberries
- 1/2 cup pecans, chopped and toasted
- 1/4 cup chopped fresh parsley
- 1/4 cup crumbled feta cheese (optional)
- 2 tablespoons extra virgin olive oil
- 1 tablespoon balsamic vinegar
- 1 tablespoon maple syrup or honey
- Salt and pepper to taste

Instructions:
1. In a medium saucepan, combine the farro and water or vegetable broth. Bring to a boil, then reduce the heat to low, cover, and simmer for 25-30 minutes, or until the farro is tender but still slightly chewy.

2. Once the farro is cooked, drain any excess liquid and transfer it to a large mixing bowl to cool.

3. In a small bowl, whisk together the extra virgin olive oil, balsamic vinegar, maple syrup or honey, salt, and pepper to make the dressing.

4. Add the dried cranberries, toasted pecans, chopped fresh parsley, and crumbled feta cheese (if using) to the bowl with the cooked farro.

5. Pour the dressing over the farro salad ingredients and toss gently to coat.

6. Taste and adjust the seasoning as needed, adding more salt and pepper if desired.

7. Serve the farro salad with cranberries and pecans immediately as a delicious and satisfying side dish or light meal.

This farro salad with cranberries and pecans is a wonderful combination of sweet, savory, and nutty flavors. It's packed with nutrients and makes for a hearty and satisfying dish that's perfect for lunch, dinner, or potlucks. Enjoy!

104. Cucumber and dill salad

Ingredients:
- 2 large cucumbers, thinly sliced
- 1/4 cup thinly sliced red onion
- 2 tablespoons chopped fresh dill
- 1/4 cup apple cider vinegar
- 2 tablespoons extra virgin olive oil
- 1 tablespoon honey or maple syrup (optional, for added sweetness)
- Salt and pepper to taste

Instructions:

1. In a large mixing bowl, combine the thinly sliced cucumbers, sliced red onion, and chopped fresh dill.

2. In a small bowl, whisk together the apple cider vinegar, extra virgin olive oil, honey or maple syrup (if using), salt, and pepper to make the dressing.

3. Pour the dressing over the cucumber mixture in the bowl.

4. Toss the cucumber and dill salad gently to coat the ingredients evenly with the dressing.

5. Taste and adjust the seasoning as needed, adding more salt and pepper if desired.

6. Cover the bowl with plastic wrap or transfer the salad to an airtight container, and refrigerate for at least 30 minutes to allow the flavors to meld together.

7. Serve the cucumber and dill salad chilled as a refreshing and light side dish or accompaniment to grilled meats or seafood.

This cucumber and dill salad is crisp, refreshing, and bursting with flavor. The combination of crunchy cucumbers, tangy red onion, and fragrant dill creates a delightful salad that's perfect for summer picnics, barbecues, or any time you're craving a light and healthy dish. Enjoy!

105. Spinach salad with mandarin oranges

Ingredients:
- 6 cups fresh baby spinach leaves
- 1 can (11 ounces) mandarin oranges, drained
- 1/4 cup sliced almonds, toasted
- 1/4 cup crumbled feta cheese (optional)
- 1/4 cup red onion, thinly sliced
- 2 tablespoons extra virgin olive oil
- 2 tablespoons balsamic vinegar
- 1 tablespoon honey or maple syrup
- Salt and pepper to taste

Instructions:
1. In a large salad bowl, combine the fresh baby spinach leaves, drained mandarin oranges, toasted sliced almonds, crumbled feta cheese (if using), and thinly sliced red onion.

2. In a small bowl, whisk together the extra virgin olive oil, balsamic vinegar, honey or maple syrup, salt, and pepper to make the dressing.

3. Pour the dressing over the spinach salad ingredients in the bowl.

4. Toss the spinach salad gently to coat the ingredients evenly with the dressing.

5. Taste and adjust the seasoning as needed, adding more salt and pepper if desired.

6. Serve the spinach salad with mandarin oranges immediately as a delicious and nutritious side dish or light meal.

This spinach salad with mandarin oranges is both refreshing and satisfying. The combination of tender spinach leaves, sweet mandarin oranges, crunchy almonds, and tangy dressing creates a flavorful and vibrant salad that's perfect for any occasion. Enjoy!

106. Green bean and almond salad

Ingredients:
- 1 pound fresh green beans, trimmed
- 1/4 cup sliced almonds, toasted
- 2 tablespoons chopped fresh parsley
- 2 tablespoons extra virgin olive oil
- 1 tablespoon lemon juice
- 1 clove garlic, minced
- Salt and pepper to taste

Instructions:
1. Bring a pot of salted water to a boil. Add the green beans and cook until tender-crisp, about 3-4 minutes.

2. Drain the green beans and immediately transfer them to a bowl of ice water to stop the cooking process. Once cooled, drain again and pat dry with paper towels.

3. In a large mixing bowl, combine the blanched green beans, toasted sliced almonds, and chopped fresh parsley.

4. In a small bowl, whisk together the extra virgin olive oil, lemon juice, minced garlic, salt, and pepper to make the dressing.

5. Pour the dressing over the green bean and almond salad ingredients in the bowl.

6. Toss the salad gently to coat the ingredients evenly with the dressing.

7. Taste and adjust the seasoning as needed, adding more salt and pepper if desired.

8. Serve the green bean and almond salad immediately as a delicious and nutritious side dish or light meal.

This green bean and almond salad is fresh, crunchy, and bursting with flavor. It's a perfect accompaniment to grilled meats or seafood, or as a standalone dish for a light and healthy lunch. Enjoy!

107. Quinoa salad with cranberries and pecans

Ingredients:
- 1 cup quinoa, rinsed
- 2 cups water or vegetable broth
- 1/2 cup dried cranberries
- 1/2 cup chopped pecans, toasted
- 1/4 cup chopped fresh parsley
- 2 green onions, thinly sliced
- 2 tablespoons extra virgin olive oil
- 2 tablespoons balsamic vinegar
- 1 tablespoon maple syrup or honey
- Salt and pepper to taste

Instructions:

1. In a medium saucepan, combine the quinoa and water or vegetable broth. Bring to a boil, then reduce the heat to low, cover, and simmer for 15-20 minutes, or until the quinoa is cooked and the liquid is absorbed. Remove from heat and let it cool.

2. In a large mixing bowl, combine the cooked quinoa, dried cranberries, toasted chopped pecans, chopped fresh parsley, and thinly sliced green onions.

3. In a small bowl, whisk together the extra virgin olive oil, balsamic vinegar, maple syrup or honey, salt, and pepper to make the dressing.

4. Pour the dressing over the quinoa salad ingredients in the bowl.

5. Toss the salad gently to coat the ingredients evenly with the dressing.

6. Taste and adjust the seasoning as needed, adding more salt and pepper if desired.

7. Serve the quinoa salad with cranberries and pecans immediately as a delicious and nutritious side dish or light meal.

This quinoa salad with cranberries and pecans is both flavorful and satisfying. It's packed with protein, fiber, and healthy fats, making it a perfect option for a nutritious lunch or dinner. Enjoy!

108. Chickpea salad with tomatoes and parsley

Ingredients:
- 2 cans (15 ounces each) chickpeas (garbanzo beans), drained and rinsed
- 1 pint cherry tomatoes, halved
- 1/4 cup chopped fresh parsley
- 1/4 cup red onion, finely chopped
- 2 tablespoons extra virgin olive oil
- 2 tablespoons lemon juice
- 1 clove garlic, minced
- Salt and pepper to taste

Instructions:

1. In a large mixing bowl, combine the drained and rinsed chickpeas, halved cherry tomatoes, chopped fresh parsley, and finely chopped red onion.

2. In a small bowl, whisk together the extra virgin olive oil, lemon juice, minced garlic, salt, and pepper to make the dressing.

3. Pour the dressing over the chickpea salad ingredients in the bowl.

4. Toss the salad gently to coat the ingredients evenly with the dressing.

5. Taste and adjust the seasoning as needed, adding more salt and pepper if desired.

6. Let the chickpea salad sit for at least 15 minutes to allow the flavors to meld together.

7. Serve the chickpea salad with tomatoes and parsley immediately as a delicious and nutritious side dish or light meal.

This chickpea salad with tomatoes and parsley is packed with protein, fiber, and vitamins, making it a healthy and satisfying option for lunch or dinner. It's easy to make and bursting with fresh flavors. Enjoy!

109. Lentil salad with lemon vinaigrette

Ingredients:
For the salad:
- 1 cup dried green or brown lentils, rinsed
- 3 cups water or vegetable broth
- 1/2 cup diced red bell pepper
- 1/2 cup diced cucumber
- 1/4 cup finely chopped red onion
- 1/4 cup chopped fresh parsley
- Salt and pepper to taste

For the lemon vinaigrette:
- 1/4 cup extra virgin olive oil
- 2 tablespoons fresh lemon juice
- 1 teaspoon Dijon mustard
- 1 clove garlic, minced
- Salt and pepper to taste

Instructions:

1. In a medium saucepan, combine the lentils and water or vegetable broth. Bring to a boil, then reduce the heat to low, cover, and simmer for 20-25 minutes, or until the lentils are tender but still hold their shape. Drain any excess liquid and let the lentils cool.

2. In a large mixing bowl, combine the cooked lentils, diced red bell pepper, diced cucumber, chopped red onion, and chopped fresh parsley.

3. In a small bowl, whisk together the extra virgin olive oil, fresh lemon juice, Dijon mustard, minced garlic, salt, and pepper to make the lemon vinaigrette.

4. Pour the lemon vinaigrette over the lentil salad ingredients in the bowl.

5. Toss the salad gently to coat the ingredients evenly with the dressing.

6. Taste and adjust the seasoning as needed, adding more salt and pepper if desired.

7. Let the lentil salad sit for at least 15 minutes to allow the flavors to meld together.

8. Serve the lentil salad with lemon vinaigrette immediately as a delicious and nutritious side dish or light meal.

This lentil salad with lemon vinaigrette is hearty, flavorful, and packed with protein and fiber. It's perfect for a light lunch or dinner, and it can be made ahead of time and stored in the refrigerator for easy meal prep. Enjoy!

110. Caprese salad with tomatoes, basil, and mozzarella

Ingredients:

- 2 large tomatoes, sliced
- 1 ball fresh mozzarella cheese, sliced
- Fresh basil leaves
- Extra virgin olive oil
- Balsamic glaze (optional)
- Salt and pepper to taste

Instructions:

1. Arrange the tomato slices and mozzarella slices alternately on a serving plate.

2. Tuck fresh basil leaves between the tomato and mozzarella slices.

3. Drizzle extra virgin olive oil over the salad.

4. Optionally, drizzle balsamic glaze over the salad for extra flavor.

5. Season with salt and pepper to taste.

6. Serve immediately as a refreshing and flavorful appetizer or side dish.

This Caprese salad celebrates the flavors of summer with ripe tomatoes, creamy mozzarella cheese, and fragrant basil. It's a light and elegant dish that's perfect for any occasion. Enjoy!

111. Orzo salad with feta and olives

Ingredients:
- 1 cup orzo pasta
- 1/4 cup extra virgin olive oil
- 2 tablespoons red wine vinegar
- 1 clove garlic, minced
- 1 teaspoon dried oregano
- Salt and pepper to taste
- 1 cup cherry tomatoes, halved
- 1/2 cup cucumber, diced
- 1/4 cup red onion, finely chopped
- 1/4 cup Kalamata olives, pitted and sliced
- 1/4 cup crumbled feta cheese
- 2 tablespoons chopped fresh parsley

Instructions:
1. Cook the orzo pasta according to the package instructions until al dente. Drain and rinse under cold water to cool.

2. In a small bowl, whisk together the extra virgin olive oil, red wine vinegar, minced garlic, dried oregano, salt, and pepper to make the dressing.

3. In a large mixing bowl, combine the cooked and cooled orzo pasta, halved cherry tomatoes, diced cucumber, finely chopped red onion, sliced Kalamata olives, crumbled feta cheese, and chopped fresh parsley.

4. Pour the dressing over the orzo salad ingredients in the bowl.

5. Toss the salad gently to coat the ingredients evenly with the dressing.

6. Taste and adjust the seasoning as needed, adding more salt and pepper if desired.

7. Let the orzo salad sit for at least 15 minutes to allow the flavors to meld together.

8. Serve the orzo salad with feta and olives immediately as a delicious and satisfying side dish or light meal.

This orzo salad with feta and olives is packed with Mediterranean flavors and makes for a refreshing and nutritious dish. It's perfect for picnics, barbecues, or as a light lunch or dinner option. Enjoy!

As we reach the end of **Nourishing Nephrons: A Culinary Guide for Chronic Kidney Disease Stage 3**, we hope you've found inspiration, empowerment, and above all, delicious ways to support your kidney health journey. Managing Stage 3 CKD can present its challenges, but with the right nutrition strategies and culinary know-how, you can take control of your diet and savor every bite along the way.

In these pages, we've explored the importance of mindful eating, understanding the role of nutrients in kidney health, and how to navigate dietary restrictions without compromising on flavor or variety. From nutrient-packed breakfasts to satisfying dinners and everything in between, each recipe has been carefully crafted to nourish your body and delight your palate.

Remember, this cookbook is not just about what you can't eat; it's about celebrating the abundance of wholesome, kidney-friendly ingredients that can enhance your meals and improve your overall well-being. It's about embracing creativity in the kitchen and discovering the joy of cooking with purpose.

As you continue your journey with Stage 3 CKD, we encourage you to experiment with these recipes, adapt them to your taste preferences, and share them with loved ones. And always remember, you are not alone. There is a community of individuals facing similar challenges, supporting each other, and finding strength in shared experiences.

Thank you for allowing Nourishing Nephrons to be a part of your culinary adventure. May these recipes bring you comfort, nourishment, and a renewed sense of vitality as you navigate life with Stage 3 CKD. Here's to your health and the joy of savoring every moment, one delicious dish at a time.